Reinventing Your Nursing Career:

A Handbook for Success in the Age of Managed Care

Michael Newell, RN, MSN, CCM
Principal
Managed Care Consultants
Merchantville, New Jersey

Mario Pinardo
President
Achievement Dynamics Institute, Inc.
Cherry Hill, New Jersey

AN ASPEN PUBLICATION®
Aspen Publishers, Inc.
Gaithersburg, Maryland
1998

Library of Congress Cataloging-in-Publication Data

Newell, Michael.
Reinventing your nursing career: a handbook for success in the
age of managed care / Michael Newell, Mario Pinardo.
p. cm.
Includes bibliographical references and index ·
ISBN 0-8342-1007-X (paper)
1. Nursing—Vocational guidance.   2. Nursing—Effect of managed care on.
3. Case Management.   I. Pinardo, Mario.   II. Title.
[DNLM: 1. Economics, Nursing—United States.   2. Nursing Services—
organization & administration—United States.   3. Managed Care Programs—
organization & administration—United States.   WY 77 N546r   1997]
RT82.N45   1997
610.73'06'9—DC21
DNLM/DLC
for Library of Congress
97-30346
CIP

Orders: (800) 638-8437
Customer Service: (800) 234-1660

About Aspen Publishers • For more than 35 years, Aspen has been a
leading professional publisher in a variety of disciplines. Aspen's vast information
resources are available in both print and electronic formats. We are committed
to providing the highest quality information available in the most appropriate
format for our customers. Visit Aspen's Internet site for more information
resources, directories, articles, and a searchable version of Aspen's full catalog,
including the most recent publications: **http://www.aspenpub.com**
Aspen Publishers, Inc. • The hallmark of quality in publishing
Member of the worldwide Wolters Kluwer group.

Editorial Resources: Kathleen Ruby
Library of Congress Catalog Card Number: 97-30346
ISBN: 0-8342-1007-X

Printed in the United States of America

1 2 3 4 5

Contents

Foreword

Only 20 years ago, the majority of American nurses worked in a hospital-dominated environment where they could expect security, automatic rewards, and support in their professional practice from their employers. That comfortable world has long since been scrambled by managed care and an onslaught of evanescent redesigns and restructurings. Now nurses are on their own in a tumultuous health care marketplace that seethes with competition and conflict, angst, and uncertainty. While these changes are accomplished by limitless opportunities, only those who are prepared will be able to take advantage of them.

My relationship with one of this book's authors, Mike Newell, spans those 20 years. We initially worked together at an urban teaching center as nurses engaged in traditional hospital roles, caring for many of the same patients. Mike reentered my life some time later, bursting with the energy of one who had learned to read and ride every change in health care to build a successful career. As a thinker, educator, lecturer, and colleague, Mike has moved in visionary circles to guide nurses toward building their own careers. With his proven track record as author of a previous book on case management, Mike has joined Mario Pinardo, an expert on professional development, to write *Reinventing Your Nursing Career: A Handbook for Success in the Age of Managed Care*. These two authors are well-matched to guide nurses in their professional journey.

This book is for nurses who wish to prepare for the future. It offers timely advice within a historical perspective so that nurses can redefine and reposition themselves for successful careers. It reflects a new paradigm that encourages nurses to break away from the outdated notions and restrictive institutions that previously defined their worth. Nurses can take control of their careers, but they must know themselves. The authors lead nurses through a self-discovery process to strengthen themselves as individuals and professionals.

At the same time, this book is a very practical manual for career enhancement. The authors provide practitioners with an orderly formula for identifying the values and goals that drive a successful professional life. The authors present a methodology for refining and acquiring skills marketable in contemporary and future practice settings.

From my vantage in a 10-year-old media company that provides career advice to almost a quarter of the RNs in the United States, I have watched nurses' mixed and sometimes frantic responses to current changes in health care. Many have become paralyzed by the realities of lost jobs and involuntary shifts in their employment situations. At the same time, a new breed of health professionals—renaissance nurses—has emerged to thrive with every change. This book provides admission to this very special group. I believe that nurses who follow the instructions within these pages will have an opportunity to become better practitioners and more marketable professionals. Armed with a renewed sense of worth and career readiness, they will be better able to fashion a renaissance in health care.

Robert Hess, PhD, RN
Editor and Corporate Director of Continuing Education
Nursing Spectrum

Preface

The current environment of health care is akin to the industrial revolution of 150 years ago. New computer, communications, imaging, genetics, fiber optics, and pharmaceutical technologies have combined with social forces that demand better service at lower costs. In the previous revolution, farmers and skilled craftspeople were displaced by machinery, and great enterprises emerged to mass-produce goods and services. The resulting displacement of families, the increased complexity of society, and the growing risks of emerging business systems led to dark tragedies as well as spectacular triumphs.

Health care is moving from a nonprofit, single-provider, fee-for-service model to a giant enterprise that is connected by computers and prepaid by employers and government. This shift demands new skills and practices from all health care workers. Nurses are the largest group of health providers in the nation—they are certain to feel the biggest impact from these changes.

For many years, nurses have been looking for ways to care for patients away from the hospital setting. Due to the current changes in the health care system, the need for this strategy and others has become more acute. This book is designed to educate nurses about why the health care system is changing, so they can use the information to reinvent their career path in a way that fulfills their professional as well as personal needs. Most self-help books tend to be anecdotal, serving up inspiring stories rather than hard facts. Although this book is not an academic text, we have tried to provide a framework for viewing the new realities of health care, some self-evaluation tools, and some references for those who want to explore further. The journey of personal and professional self-discovery cannot be mapped out like a clinical procedure manual. Herein are tools that can be used to assist every practitioner in assessing his or her current career, and a step-by-step guide to enrich one's personal relationships and professional practice.

Whereas the short-term future of health care appears grave, the long-term prognosis for nurses appears to be good. Nurses are in a perfect position to fit in to the newly emerging system. If they can take the initiative to develop the skills, attitudes, and vision that the new system will require, they can assist their employers in meeting the demands of a public that expects the best health care in the world.

Not all nurses will fit in to the new corporate model of health delivery. However, there is an increasing preference by consumers to seek out services that provide what industrialized medicine has not been able to provide: a sense of meaning, a sense of connectedness, and help with healing.

This book is designed to assist nurses and other health care practitioners who need to know more about how and why the system works the way it does, and how they can realize their personal and professional vision about what health care can be.

Acknowledgments ___

Thank you to my wife Nadia, and our children Michael, Domenica, and Catherine for their support.

Michael Newell

———⊰⊙⊙⊙⊱———

This book is dedicated to all people who wake up and feel it is time to grab hold and take charge of who they are and what they want. Sometimes, it is necessary to give permission to make personal life changes that complement values and dreams, and to drive the changes in life in a direction with positive, exciting results.

And a thank you to my wonderful wife Reneé and daughter Maria for their unwavering patience and love and Francis E. Sinatra for his expertise and help in the development of this manuscript.

Mario Pinardo

Part I

The Dynamics of a Dis-Integrating Health Care System

INTRODUCTION

The first part of this book is designed to assist nurses in understanding the changes in finance, technology, and public expectations that are driving many of the changes in the health care industry. These changes have been coming for a long time, but they are accelerating rather than slowing down, causing disorientation for health care providers, insurance companies, government regulators, politicians, and patients alike.

Some of the incentives of the old system will go away as providers are forced to be more efficient. New ethical and legal situations are arising as the work force is reduced, companies merge, and the responsibility of making health care decisions and payment decisions changes. These chapters are meant to provide a sophisticated overview rather than an academic treatment of what is happening, why, and what you can do now.

Chapter 1 reviews the recent history of the financing of health care, why the system costs so much, and how health services are paid for. The concepts of risk-bearing contracts, reengineering, and the impact of technology are discussed. The emphasis is on understanding how the different parts of the system interact, so that those in the health care field who are planning their futures can anticipate some of the trends. The issue of the value of services and how services and value are linked in the minds of consumers is very important.

Chapter 2 looks at how nurses see themselves and how they *should* see their value in the future. Nurses must begin to give themselves more

1

credit and learn how to demonstrate the value of the services they provide. Some of the more recent trends in new practice settings for nurses are described here.

Chapter 3 discusses the issue of value from the viewpoint of the corporation and others in the health system. All of us need to have our own clear definition of health, if we are going to design careers that are congruent with the practice setting we choose. **Chapter 4** discusses the skill sets necessitated by some of these new settings and presents a skill matrix that can lead to some new concepts for nurses who need to rethink their current personal and professional situation.

Chapter 5 discusses the latest nursing subspecialty, case management. If health care is going to address the real needs of most patients, then case management makes sense. Case management demands mature, skilled nurses who communicate well with patients, providers, and peers. It requires creative thinking and the ability to coach and counsel patients and their families in ways that most nurses have been prevented from doing in the physician-dominated settings of hospitals, nursing homes, and ambulatory care.

1

Future Directions of the Health Care System

The business of health care (or the practice of medicine and nursing) in the age of managed care is a titanic fireworks exhibition that is *just beginning*. The increased consolidation of hospitals, physicians, nursing homes, and health maintenance organizations (HMOs) elicits wonder from the crowd of onlookers: investors, regulators, practitioners, and John and Jane Q. Public. The rockets are streaking skyward, promising the most beautiful arc to the heavens, the biggest bang, the most dazzling cascade of services to thrill subscribers, patients, employers, and health care providers alike.

This fireworks display foreshadows more sparkles than heat, more smoke and cinders than illumination, more bombs than bouquets. Society is giving its health system to the entrepreneurs in the twofold belief that (1) these entrepreneurs can bring the best value for the dollars spent and (2) the government is not the best administrator of services that ultimately affect the common good. These beliefs, whether everyone agrees with them or not, will determine the efficiency and probably the effectiveness of medical services. Like stray fireworks that plunge into the onlooking crowd, however, health care systems that

3

are not carefully planned will cause chaos and pandemonium that will hurt many.

The United States has approximately 950,000 hospital beds. The projection is that within five years, the number will be reduced to 425,000. At 4.2 full-time–equivalent positions (FTEs) per bed, these figures indicate that about 1.8 million hospital workers will be displaced from their jobs.[1] Half of these will be nurses.

The news is not all bad. Because people are living longer and the number of those entering the profession of nursing is decreasing, anyone who wants to work in nursing will be able to work in the field. Nurses may not work in the setting or for the pay and professional advancement level that they would like, however. Hospitals may not be the main setting for the practicing professional nurse of the future, for example, but there are opportunities in other settings. The fields of case management, public health, ambulatory care, long-term care, and home care are all expanding. Opportunities for niche practices focused on groups of patients who have chronic or special needs are emerging daily.

The situation for physicians is more problematic. The HMOs already have decided that they need only so many physicians per 1,000 covered lives (the number of people who belong to an HMO), and many more of them will be primary care physicians (PCPs) than specialty physicians. Of the 625,000 practicing physicians, the HMOs will have use for only about 325,000, once 90 percent of the population is under a managed health care plan. That HMO penetration rate (i.e., the percentage of subscribers in an HMO) was 26 percent by the end of 1995[2] but will rise very steeply as Medicare and Medicaid convert to managed health care across the United States. Specialists, including orthopaedists, anesthetists, and cardiologists, are already experiencing decreases in their referrals and their fee structures. Many physicians are banding together in huge specialty group practices to protect their business. Some are talking about unionization. It remains to be seen if any of these strategies will work.

REASONS FOR CHANGE IN THE HEALTH CARE SYSTEM

Government officials have been talking about changing the health care system for a long time. The employers who are largely paying for health insurance started the discussion, and the media fueled it with stories of how many dollars are spent, how much physicians make, how many people are uninsured, and so forth. The prospect of paying the enormous costs of health insurance and health care out of their pockets frightens people. They know that without access to insurance, they risk the catastrophe of being denied care, receiving substandard care, and being ruined financially. The reasons for the demise of the old system have to do with cost shifting, which drove up the price of health coverage paid by employers; the staggering costs of entitlements (e.g., Medicare, Medicaid, and Social Security Disability); and a change in the public perception of the value of the health care rendered.

Cost Shifting

In the area of health care costs, the term *cost shifting* means that the provider shifts the cost of care from one type of payer or patient to another. Hospitals shifted the costs associated with care of the indigent, uncollectable bills, and lower rates paid by Medicare and Medicaid patients to private insurance companies. These indemnity insurance plans (i.e., the typical group health or Blue Cross plans) paid the higher charges but made up for their increased costs by shifting their costs to the consumers of their products—mostly the employers who paid for employee health insurance.

This situation was ripe for the growth of managed care organizations (MCOs), both the preferred provider organizations (PPOs), which have a select panel of physicians and facilities that provide care at a discounted rate, and HMOs, which provide care at a fixed premium with no deductibles as long as the subscriber goes to the approved panel of providers. Although MCOs had been around since the early 1970s, they had not become common in most parts of the United States. Now the accelerated shift in costs, caused in part by the fact that MCOs paid a discounted rate, placed the traditional health insurance carriers in a difficult position. As they raised their premiums to cover the cost shifts and "medical inflation" (rising costs brought about by the greater use of technology and higher provider fees), they lost business because their rates were too high.

The Clinton Administration moved to do something about this by developing a health plan, but the plan was too complex, tried to please too many constituents who liked the old way (e.g., physicians, hospitals, the elderly), and threatened the insurance industry at its very foundation. (If the cash flow from health policies disappeared overnight by legislative decree, some feared that it would lead to a collapse of the entire U.S. economy.) The natural debate regarding the Clinton Health Plan did give the insurance companies time to plan a shift in their strategy, however. Many have either left the health policy business (most of the smaller firms) or have tried to shift their subscribers into the newer HMO plans.

Entitlements

The Social Security, Medicare, and Medicaid programs were originally conceived as a social safety net for the elderly and for those too frail or too sick to hold a job. The good news about the health of the nation is that more people are living longer than was anticipated. The bad news is that most of these people require health care services and money to sustain their life, and the financial burden of meeting their needs will severely strain the nation's ability to sustain itself.

The federal government has taken steps within the past several years to decrease entitlements, the government benefits to which those who are sick or old are "entitled," no matter what the cost. These entitlements have increased with the rise in the consumer index, which is calculated on the basis of the rate of inflation and the cost of living. In one effort to reduce entitlements, the government has made the entry into the system more difficult, raising the standard of eligibility for disability benefits and insisting that all businesses make their facilities accessible to the disabled. The passage of the Americans with Disabilities Act to promote employment among all those who may not have had access to work because of their disabilities contributed to this effort.[3]

Medicare

In 1995, the Medicare program cost the federal treasury approximately $190 billion, covering about 35 million people. It has been estimated that the costs will increase about 10 percent annually to $294 billion by the year 2000.[4] The Medicare system tried prospective payment for hospitals, relative value scales for payment of physician services, and other schemes to attempt to control the flow of dollars out of the treasury, all with little effect. The problem is that the government was actually paying for medical care rather than health care. Because the medical model is centered on doctors and hospitals and always has a cure as its ultimate goal, it consumes far more resources than those required by the health care model.

Federal efforts to implement cost savings often encounter schemes to increase utilization that are launched by those who know how to manipulate the system. For example, a federal attempt to lower costs by discharging patients from hospitals sooner met with the rise in subacute services. Patients in subacute care do not require hospital care, with its emphasis on diagnostic procedures and invasive treatments; but they do need skilled nursing care and rehabilitation. These patients are usually elderly, may be deconditioned, and often have other problems that interfere with intensive (five hours per day or greater) rehabilitative services. Medicare pays for up to 100 days of subacute care, with little prospective or concurrent utilization review of the need for the care. Consequently, subacute care, both in hospitals and nursing homes, has grown enormously in recent years, with little benefit over the old way (continued inpatient hospital care) seen for patients.

Those on Medicare qualify for the entitlement because they are elderly or disabled. Chronic, incurable, disabling diseases come with age. A person's state of health changes over time with environmental exposures, stress, poor health habits, and lack of social and family support. Coping with the impairments brought about by physical deterioration mandates that patients and their families learn to limit the consequence of the disease, take steps to adapt to its limitations, and maintain an optimal level of physical functioning. This is a great deal of work, but pretending there is a cure just drives up the cost and leads to frustration for everyone.

Medicaid

What nurses hear about Medicaid patients or experience in one-to-one clinical situations does not give an accurate picture of who gets Medicaid and why. The federal and state governments share the costs of the Medicaid program, but state governments must meet certain federal guidelines to be eligible for funding. The advent of the Medicaid system largely did away with many county hospitals over the years. Once hospitals saw they could make money treating the poor instead of relegating them to charity-care institutions, poor patients were welcomed to mainstream hospitals. Many cities and counties then gradually closed their public hospitals over the years. A fiscal intermediary (an insurance company that handled the claims) paid for health care on behalf of the state. Each state set benefit levels and entitlement requirements. The yearly outlay for Medicaid was $138 billion for 36 million recipients in 1995, or about $3,800 per recipient per year. This cost is projected to rise to $215 billion by the year 2000.

Approximately half of the Medicaid money is spent on nursing home care for those who are elderly and have exhausted their financial resources. Of the Medicaid recipients who are not institutionalized, about 75 percent are under the age of 21; their mothers make up most of the rest of the recipients. Medicaid, then, is a program designed to pay for care needed by our most fragile citizens. The cost, especially for long-term care, is draining the treasuries of both the federal and state governments.

Physicians and hospitals used to think of Medicaid and Medicare as very poor payers. The rates are below what providers have been accustomed to charging, and the payment is often slow, especially if the bills are not correctly submitted. Now many providers who participate in MCOs are trying to increase the number of their Medicare and Medicaid patients because the per subscriber per month payment is relatively high.

Although there are some Medicaid HMOs (only 10 percent of Medicaid recipients were enrolled in managed care plans in 1995), there is not enough experience with Medicaid managed care to indicate if it will work well with young, poor, urban populations. Health is a function of many factors, among them the quality of housing, nutrition, education, social support, and public health infrastructure (e.g., good municipal water/sewerage systems, programs for immunizations and prenatal care).

Public Perception of Value

In general, value is the perception of worth in relation to the cost. Health care services have suffered because so many people, although they understand the worth of insurance coverage, are either unwilling or unable to pay for it. (This compounds the problem of cost shifting, because the approximately 40 million U.S. citizens who have no health coverage[5] require expensive care after they get sick.) The public's perception of the value of health care services will dictate the kind of system that will eventually prevail. People must decide what they really want from the system.

One good thing about managed care is that it has exploded many of the myths about health care services that have prevailed over the years.

Myth #1: The doctor knows (what constitutes quality) best

The fee-for-service system of health care in the United States is undoubtedly the most technically proficient in the world, but it has largely overreached itself in terms of providing what it promises to most patients (i.e., a cure). Moreover, when MCOs instituted early discharges, questioned the need for extensive (and expensive) testing, and began to have PCPs direct the care of many patients, there was no observable decline in the quality of care as determined by measures of morbidity, mortality, and complication rates. Many MCOs have also ranked equal to or above fee-for-service plans in terms of patient satisfaction. The insistence of the MCOs that physicians and hospitals justify their treatment plans in advance (prospectively) and during the hospital stay (concurrently) has simply forced these providers to be more focused in their procedures and documentation.

Although physicians set themselves up as the final arbiters of quality, they unfortunately did not effectively police the members of their profession to prevent malpractice or excessive and fraudulent billing. They overlooked the perception of value by the customers (i.e., the payers and patients) for far too long. Quality, however, is a measure of value that is judged mainly by the customer. Physicians are most qualified to set the technical specifications for medical practice, but only the patient, his or her family, and the payer (i.e., the employer whose employee returns to work, the insurance company whose fiscal responsibility to its shareholders is to maintain a viable business) can judge the end product, or outcome of care.

Myth #2: High price equals good quality

Temple University Hospital is in one of the poorest sections of Philadelphia, and the surrounding neighborhood has all the social problems that come with poverty: crime, drug wars, poor housing, unemployment, family strife, alcoholism, and so forth. On any given Saturday night the emergency department (ED)

Notes

may have a half-dozen medical emergencies. Working there a few years ago, I found that the ED was not especially well equipped or staffed; however, the medical and nursing care was excellent. When there was an emergency, everyone knew what his or her role was, so there was little discussion during the emergency as to who was to do what and when. This efficiency was due partly to a sense of teamwork and community within the institution and partly to the frequency with which the staff dealt with critical situations.

There was another university hospital that had qualified as a Level I trauma center and had an excellent reputation as a center of research and innovative care; I worked there during a time of staff shortage. I saw the first emergency only after four weeks, and it was a study in pandemonium. It was impossible to tell which attending physician was directing the code. Medical students crowded around the bedside, and there was great confusion about what was to be done for the patient. The patient died.

Thus, it was clearly apparent that facilities and practitioners who have practice, training, teamwork, and motivation to do better at each encounter with the patient can provide a better quality of care at a lower cost. Better quality of care happens when practitioners communicate better with each other so as to avoid mistakes, when practitioners communicate better with patients and families, and when practitioners communicate better with payer representatives, letting them know what the treatment rationale is in a proactive way. That way the facility receives payment for what it does and need not shift the cost to someone else. Thus, better quality health care can cost less.

The CPT Manual: Rigging the Game

The providers of care (e.g., physicians, hospitals, laboratories, radiology enterprises) have long been setting the price of care and determining the meaning of quality care with little input from the customers, the purchasers, and end users of the care (e.g., employers and patients). To this day, the American Medical Association (AMA) is the sole author of *The Manual of Current Procedural Terminology* (the *CPT Manual*), which determines how components of care will be identified, defined, and billed. This book is the bible of billing. If a provider performs some service that does not fit into the coding scheme, the likelihood that an insurance company will pay for it is slim. The coding schemes are very detailed about diagnostic, technical, and surgical procedures but scant when dealing with the cognitive and counseling aspects of health care.

About 500 CPT codes are billed by nurses, but they constitute just a fraction of all the costs listed in the manual. The fee schedule that insurers have for paying for the services of nurses is markedly lower than those for the cognitive services of family physicians and internal medicine physicians. The reason these "usual and customary" (U&C) services pay so much less originates in the way that so many U&C fees were developed.

By way of illustration, Dr. Melvin Carbuncle has invented a new procedure for painlessly snipping the nosehairs of Fortune 500 executives. This procedure is completely painless, and Dr. Carbuncle has published evidence alleging that the absence of nosehairs is linked to lowered blood pressure and risk for heart attacks and stroke. The tabloid newspapers and television newsmagazines alike have crowed over this breakthrough.

Because Dr. Carbuncle is the only one to do this procedure, he set the price. In doing so, he calculated a variety of factors: the equipment he had to buy, the time he took to develop this innovation, his office overhead, his monthly mortgage payment, advice from his wife. Then he arrived at a fee for this service that he felt was reasonable. Then he increased it by 40 percent, factoring in how much the insurance company would reduce what they would pay, how much he might have to pay a collection agency to collect the balance billed to the patient, and a hassle factor. The resulting fee then became the basis, or benchmark, for the U&C fee for performing the nasal follectomy. A *CPT Manual* description of the service was later written and a code assigned.

Now Dr. Carbuncle travels widely, hosting seminars that train physicians to do nasal follectomies in one weekend. He provides them with all they need to perform the service. For a one-time fee, this entrepreneur provides the new equipment, a training video on the technique, a toll-free customer service number, and the code words used to describe the procedure. Dr. Carbuncle then relates one more important factor: his charges for the procedure. Now all other physicians who perform nasal follectomies will bill exactly the same fee. Not only that, if insurance companies or patients object to the fee, they will be treated to the ultimate argument regarding why the procedure costs what it does: *It's the usual and customary fee!*

With all the new procedures and medical gadgets that come into the market, it seems that even the President of the United States is powerless to do anything about the cost of medical care. Major health care organizations appear to be rigging the medical reimbursement game, and it is no wonder there are scant resources to pay the hands-on practitioners who give care and comfort, guidance and empathy to patients and their families. The health care system is in trouble because it has lost its sense of values. Nurses can respond to this only by being clear about what the prevailing values of health are, where they fit in, and what skills they have to bring to the equation.

THE CORPORATIZATION OF THE HEALTH CARE SYSTEM

Although the spirit of enterprise is not new to medical and health care services, it was once common for health care to be a nonprofit community service, carried out as part of the mission of religious organizations, the public health infrastructure, or even fraternal organizations. Much of the industry tended to be locally owned, small-scale (half of the hospitals in the United States have fewer than 100 beds), and not-for-profit facilities.

To Profit or Not To Profit?

The term *nonprofit* can be deceiving at times, because every organization strives to have more revenue than expenses. The distribution of that money is then a function of the corporate bylaws. In for-profit corporations, the investors receive the profits. These investors may be partners or stockholders, and their ability to influence the various actions of the corporation depends on the corporate model and profit distribution plan. Nonprofit corporations benefit the entire community. For this reason, these enterprises receive special tax benefits. Officers of the nonprofit corporation should not directly benefit from the success of the corporation, although they are often handsomely rewarded by bonus checks.

Some of the characteristics of nonprofit corporations tend to make them less efficient. A hospital that makes more money than its incurred expenses, for example, may invest in new services that are not needed. Spending money on a program of marginal benefit drives the increase in costs for all its services. The bureaucracies built to provide the marginal service fight to keep their perceived share of the institution's budget. The department head who is weak or cannot show that his or her department is pulling its weight loses resources when resources are limited, as has been the case in the last few years. As a result, the departments that are eliminated may not be the ones that deserve it.

An example would be a neonatal intensive care unit in a region that already has enough of these beds. The hospital may have started this unit to compete with a neighboring hospital before the advent of cost containment. Now the hospital is losing money, not only on the neonatal unit, but also on its pediatric inpatient admissions. The obstetricians want these beds available in case their patients have a problem. These situations make for difficult decisions for hospitals.

The consolidation and downsizing in health care have been about managing the dollars rather than managing the care. The short-term fix of reducing the number of FTEs and increasing the revenue:expenses ratio cannot continue indefinitely. Hospitals have enormous fixed costs (about 60 percent of their budgets) to maintain the buildings and beds. Many hospitals also have enormous debts remaining from past building projects. Reengineering the business processes and consolidating operations have been used with various rates of success.

There was a belief in the 1980s that market competition would drive down the cost of health care. The opposite happened because the laws of supply and demand do not rule health care. Huge sums of money were spent on mostly high-technology equipment and services that actually increased health care costs. Additionally, where there are too many programs of a certain type (e.g., coronary artery bypass graft surgery or neonatal intensive care units), providers do not get enough practice to keep the program functioning optimally. Good health service programs get to be good from training and stay good through practice.

For-Profit Perks

Nominally, for-profit enterprises are not beholden to the community with which they do business. They take their profits and distribute them to their investors or stockholders, who may be on the other side of the world. The advantage to the community is that the management of a for-profit enterprise is often efficient. Old and lazy habits are tossed out. Correct procedure is emphasized because the organization tends to focus on the customers' real needs. People expect more from a for-profit company than from a nonprofit company. Therefore, the technical standard of care tends to rise as for-profit providers begin to gain influence in health care delivery.

The downside is that the for-profit hospital is not beholden to the community. If the hospital does not make economic sense, does not turn a profit, it will close. Some for-profit hospitals have bought and will continue to buy nonprofit hospitals just to close them. Buying out weak competitors is one strategy to increase profits. Hospitals in marginal neighborhoods and rural areas are likely to feel the brunt of this change.

THE CONCEPT OF RISK-BEARING CONTRACTS

In a risk-bearing arrangement, one party agrees to take care of the expenses of another who pays a fee or premium for the first party to assume the risk that the second party will have such expenses. Thus, an HMO takes on the risk for all medical expenses spelled out in the insurance contract with the subscriber. HMOs may ask physicians, hospitals, or integrated delivery systems to take on this risk with them. In return, the HMO collects the fees, processes the claims, and performs marketing and quality assurance functions.

The provider receives a certain amount of money per subscriber per month, also called a capitated arrangement. The scale varies according to the services to be provided and the age and sex of the subscriber. A PCP may get $12 per subscriber per month, for example, whether the subscriber seeks care at the office or not. (This is the industry average in Philadelphia.) The hospital may get $40 per subscriber per month, but be required to provide all the services that the subscriber needs if hospitalized. This scheme is supposed to encourage providers to be efficient and effective in the care that they render.

The risk-sharing arrangement forces providers to be more careful about how they treat covered patients. The old scattershot approach to diagnosis and try-everything treatment plans common in fee-for-service situations cause the provider to lose money under such an arrangement. Provider organizations must be much more careful in their allocation of resources if they are going to survive in the age of managed care. This can be good for nurses.

Nurses are cost-effective providers of care in many settings. Nurse practitioners tend to take more time to interview patients than physicians do, but order fewer diagnostic tests, recommend less medication, and encourage more self-management by patients of their (usually chronic) conditions. In hospitals, nurses are more cost-effective employees than are unlicensed assistive personnel, because nurses have a better work ethic, make fewer mistakes, and do not require nearly as much supervision.

Types of Risk

The provider organizations and insurance companies enter into agreements, both accepting the risk that they may lose money on the delivery of health care services for a fixed dollar amount. Insurance companies try to predict and limit their losses by calculating the degree of risk for a given population of health care subscribers, or covered lives (this is called "underwriting"). Actuaries estimate future expenses based on historical utilization and costs for each service, taking into account such factors as subscriber age and sex, the economic class of the insured members, general economic trends, and the benefit levels of the proposed insurance/risk plan. Epidemiologic data on the incidence and prevalence of disease for the covered population per 1,000 lives, adjusted for subscribers' age demographic, are used to predict the types of services that subscribers will require, the level of reserves that the insurer will need to pay for those services, and the prices and types of services that the provider will be expected to administer.

Actuarial Risks

Actuaries are highly paid professionals who use complex statistical models to predict risk. They look at the historical use and costs of services, severity adjustment data, and apply certain assumptions to model risk for the unique set of subscribers whom they are assisting. Although the figures they produce are treated as gospel, the data are highly dependent on the accuracy of the historical use data, vagaries in the severity adjustment models (which are far from coherent), and other assumptions about restrictions on the benefits of the health insurance plan.

Business Risks

Organizations that take on risk, whether they be insurance companies, capitated single providers, or integrated health care delivery systems, are faced not only with the newly accepted risks, but also with the normal risks of doing business. These risks center around such activities as

- signing up subscribers (The HMOs have long been accused of selecting subscribers with the least risk to use services—"cherry picking.")
- assessing the market (the demand for the organization's services at any given time)
- efficiently providing service
- collecting data on what services were provided
- determining the cost of providing the service

As each organization is challenged continuously to improve the quality of the service and decrease the price, the ability of the organization to learn and improve comes under the category of a business risk.

Legal Risks

A health care organization takes on many legal risks. Will the care be efficient and effective? Will there be lawsuits? Will the organization measure up to regulator and certification expectations? These legal risks must be managed in a proactive way.

Payers (i.e., insurance companies and large employers) have their own obligations to report quality. The Health Plan Employer Data and Information Set (HEDIS) was instituted as a way for large employers to compare the quality of services that HMOs provide. The data include such information as the timing of children's immunizations, the number of cervical cancer screenings, and other information thought to indicate the quality of preventive services.

HMOs have their own sets of stakeholders: federal and state regulators, consumer groups, politicians, investors, physicians and other providers, subscribers and their employers. Their own accrediting body, the National Commission for Quality Assurance (NCQA), is pushing the HEDIS as a fundamental quality and accreditation measure. NCQA needs patient-specific data concerning member satisfaction, improvement in health status, effectiveness in comparison with competitors regionally and nationally, and other process indicators of quality. The building blocks for these data come from the clinician's ability to value, understand, and collect meaningful information, as well as to act on the results of data analysis in order to benefit the HMO and, in turn, the HMO's customers.

Further legal risks involve the quality of care itself. Does the patient have access to appropriate care? Denials of care and issues around responsiveness to patient and family needs can lead to legal actions that are expensive to defend and erode the credibility of the organization. In hospitals, legal risks commonly arise in connection with infection control; incidents involving injuries or potential injuries to patients, employees, and visitors; and the credentialing of clinical providers within the organization. Additional legal risks accompany the contracts that providers sign with MCOs. The specifications of the contract may unfairly obligate the provider organization to deliver services· that were not anticipated, or subscriber expectations may not match the provider organization's perception of the extent of services to be rendered under the capitated contract.

Nurses as Risk Managers

If they are properly trained and have the support in place to assist them, nurses can be very effective risk managers. Nurses understand the health care system and the motivations of most of the participants. In most acute care hospital settings, nurses are now managing legal risks. The financial risks of managing groups of subscribers in a capitated system hinge on identifying those patients who are most likely to require extensive health care services, or those who are not likely to fare well in the system. These high-risk subscribers include the frail elderly, those with depression or other psychiatric diseases, those who assess their own state of health as poor, and those with long-standing chronic debilitating diseases (e.g., multiple sclerosis). Many organizations have used case management as a technique to manage the risk of excessive resource utilization with certain subsets of patients. Others are field-testing additional disease state management strategies to manage chronic conditions across the continuum of care.

Quality improvement initiatives by risk-bearing provider organizations will be focusing on better managing the risks of providing care. The projects and data collection will involve getting better information about the incidence of disease, treatment choices available, physician practice patterns, and so forth, so as to assist the actuaries with their task to predict more accurately the type and cost of services needed.

LINKAGE

To any organization that treats patients for all their health care needs, the concept of linkage is important. If the management of the patient's care is efficient and effective, no matter what the setting, the cost should go down, and the quality and patient satisfaction should go up. Because linkage requires practitioners who know about medical management, understand the workings of the health care system, have the training and socialization to be patient advocates, and are not dogmatic about solving the patient's problem, nurses are the ideal health care professionals to assist in managing patients over the entire continuum of care.

Linkage involves bringing added value to patients and other stakeholders by linking

- medical interventions to the stated needs of the patient
- the intensity of service to the most appropriate setting
- the treatment settings to each other without re-dundancies
- patients and their families to personal and com-munity resources
- the plan of care to the patient-defined needs
- the incentives for the patient and other stake-holders to the outcome of care
- providers to customers in new ways that show value to payers and patients alike

Issues related to linkage in the evolution of health care services are both strategic and operational. Risk management considerations also need to be consid-ered in program design and operation.

Strategic Linkage

A primary part of strategic linkage involves plan-ning strategies that meet customer needs (Table 1–1).

Table 1–1: Example: Identification of Customer/Stakeholder Satisfaction for a Hospital

Customers	Criteria for Judgment	Judgment

Payers
  MCOs
  Medicare
  Medicaid
  Auto insurance
  Workers'
    compensation
  Union health
    insurance
  Large employer
    health insurance
	Patient complaints
	Reputation in community
	Ease of access
	Range of services
	Location
	Physical plant
	Quality of physicians
	Billed within reasonable
	  time
	Bills properly coded
	Medical records with
	  bills
	Return phone calls?
	Able to retrieve records?
		Numerous complaints
		  concerning emergency
		  room waits
		Seen as declining
		  institution due to
		  decline in neighbor-
		  hood
		Safe parking a problem
		Need more board-
		  certified primary
		  care doctors
		Records, reports not sent
		  with bill
		Records report activity
		  that does not match
		  codes on bills
		Diagnosis codes (ICD-9)
		  and CPT codes some-
		  times incongruent

State regulators	Compliance with state
	  and Joint Commission on
	  Accreditation of Health-
	  care Organizations	

Employees	Labor relations, personal policies	
Board of trustees	Efficiency of management Reputation in community Proactive in community	
Physicians	Ease of referrals Quality of support staff Quality of specialists Prestige in community Compliance with orders	
Educational institutions	Site for training Generation of research	
Suppliers	Accessibility Bills paid on time	

In order to plan a strategy for success as individuals and as team members of a provider organization, nurses need to answer three basic questions:

1. Who are their customers?
2. By what criteria do the customers judge them?
3. What is the customers' judgment?

The nurses should rank customers (i.e., stakeholders) with respect to their power over the nurses' success. Thus, paying customers, those who pay individual salaries or organizational charges, are the most important stakeholders. Other customers include those who may influence the rate at which nurses are paid, such as supervisors who evaluate performance or patients and families who fill out satisfaction forms. Until nurses are clear on who their customers are, they cannot have a strategy to address customer concerns.

Determining the criteria by which customers judge nurses enables nurses to rank the things that need the most attention. If the most important thing to the customer is cost, then it is necessary to find a way to lower costs and make sure that the customer is aware of success in this area of endeavor. If the most important thing is quality, it is necessary to define and measure quality. Knowledge of the criteria for assessment as individuals and organizations will help nurses to improve their strategies for success.

Timely feedback from customers and other stakeholders can assist nurses in changing behaviors or programs. Nurses must link what they do to the value perceived by the customer/stakeholder. Once this link is clear, it is easier to identify the right moves to improve customer relations.

In managed care, the concept of strategic linkage means the following:

- Keep patients captured within the system; do not allow them to go to an out-of-network provider that may cost more or not be aware of the MCO's treatment algorithms.
- Show a link between the service rendered and the outcome of service.
- Show a link between the cost of service and the outcome, based on outcomes defined by the customer. Such customer-defined outcomes may include levels of disability, the cost of delivering the service, the amount of time required for treatment, and the length of time before the patient was able to return to work.
- Maintain/improve market share. When others "link" or identify an MCO as a quality provider or seek a particular individual's service as a nurse, market share increases.
- Improve physician (and other provider) and payer relations by linking the MCO to a reputation for good customer service and responsiveness.

Operational Linkage

One way to make clinical and business processes more user-friendly so that stakeholders will prefer to use particular services is through operational linkage. At the same time, an organization can link its service to quality in stakeholders' minds by eliminating redundant activities required because they were not done right the first time. This includes interviewing patients over and over as they go from one setting to another.

Linking the risks mentioned previously to a good outcome involves a repertoire of strategies:

- Complaint management to handle any subscriber/patient/family complaints about service in a way that answers the complaint incident itself and the cause for the complaint.

- Contract management. Reviewing the contract with the MCO ensures that there is no hidden cost to the provider organization for unanticipated services.
- "Demand management." Providing a toll-free telephone number for the subscriber/patient to access help for advice or information, or to expedite referrals, reduces the demand for services. This technique, using nurses who answer telephones 24 hours a day, is said to reduce costs to MCOs or provider organizations by 25 to 50 percent.[6] Some demand management programs are sponsored by the MCOs or integrated delivery systems; others may be generated by a group of physicians who have a capitated contract.

TECHNOLOGY: THE GREAT ENABLER

Technology in health care has been both a boon and a bane. Although it has enabled more precise diagnosis of anatomic conditions, payers have sometimes felt the costs to be a burden for the sometimes marginal benefits.

Severe underestimation of the real cost of technology has complicated the planning for the purchase of high-technology diagnostic equipment. The purchase of the high-technology equipment itself makes up only 20 percent of the total cost of the service. The remaining 80 percent of the real costs are in the building of an infrastructure to house the technology (e.g., masonry or shielded structures to house magnetic resonance imaging equipment); the hiring, training, and equipping of technicians to operate the technology; the service contract and upgrading of the technology; the insurance and other risk management safeguards for untoward reactions to the technology; the repeated performance of tests not done properly the first time; and the need to hospitalize the patient extra days when the technology goes "off-line."

There is a learning curve with technology. A technique that seems a miracle cure at first may later be found to be of marginal usefulness in relation to the costs of the equipment and the eventual benefit to the patient. Once the technology is introduced, however, it takes on a life of its own; physicians order the tests, or patients may demand the tests despite the absence of any real benefit.

Some habits of thought and expectation by consumers also contribute to higher than needed costs and more risk to the patient and the population as a whole. As an example, the overtreatment of commons colds, earaches, and so forth among the population, particularly with children, contributes to higher costs, the proliferation of mutant strains or bacteria, and the side effects of the drugs themselves on thousands of people.

Clinical Technology

The development of fiber-optic technology has facilitated the diagnosis and treatment of conditions that warrant surgical intervention. The ability to enter almost any body cavity cleanly and then to view, photograph, irrigate, snip, suction, take specimens for biopsy, and inflate various balloons has enabled physicians to perform procedures without hospitalizing the patient overnight or administering general anesthesia. Such procedures as magnetic resonance imaging, ultrasonography, and positron emission tomography have made it possible to view soft tissues and observe moment-to-moment changes in the body. This has expanded treatment options and requires the consumer (whether the patient or the payer) to be more conversant with the relative merits of available interventions.

It is said that 80 to 85 percent of medical interventions have no demonstrated effectiveness; that is, one type of intervention has not been shown to be more effective than another. For example, is a transurethral prostatectomy more effective than watchful waiting in a 75-year-old man with prostate disease, or are the side effects of the surgery (short-term nuances such as pain, prolonged bleeding, and possible wound infections, or long-term side effects such as incontinence and impotence) more trouble than the disease? Because so many medical procedures lack clearly demonstrated efficiency and effectiveness, payers have begun to demand outcome data on the interventions used. This has led to the widespread development of clinical or critical paths. Traditionally, most physicians made treatment recommendations based on their experience (i.e., their training, the advice of their colleagues in the same city). Now, however, the push is for evidence-based medical practice. Best-practice treatment processes are based on clinical studies, the recommendations of panels of experts, and clinical paths based on specialty society recommendations.

The availability of clinical guidelines and the emerging standardization of treatments remove some individual choices of physicians. Some see this as an advancement in the practice of medicine, because it tends to streamline the business processes of the workflow and clarify for all treatment team members the expectations for each patient on any given day as the treatment protocol progresses. Further, it is easier to observe and record variations of the response to treatment; to train new staff as to the expectations of the treatment; and to predict for the patient, family, and insurer the next steps in the treatment plan.

Business Process Technology

Advances in the efficiency of health care services are essential if individual provider organizations are to survive and meet customer needs. Greater efficiency in the business processes of patient care must become part of the improvement effort. Such efficiency includes eliminating redundant activity; properly recording the cost aspect of the care component; electronically transmitting patient information such as physicians' orders, prescriptions, and bills to the proper place and payer in a timely fashion; and having information available to off-site decision makers so that treatment decisions can be timely.

The quest for efficiency in the provision of health care services is not new. Millions of dollars have been spent to computerize physicians' offices, hospitals, and insurance companies, sometimes with disastrous results. Most computerization efforts fail because the computer vendor does not understand the business needs of the health care provider. In order to use computers to automate business processes, the design of the computer system must match the actual process needed to do the task efficiently. Backup systems and adequate training of those who are expected to run the system are essential.

Computerization

Hospitals now spend about 2 to 3 percent of their budget on computers to support the financial aspects of their operations, to enter orders, to conduct laboratory and radiologic tests, and, in some cases, to collect patient information at the bedside. By contrast, the banking industry spends 10 to 12 percent of its budget on information technology that helps to speed transactions and track large amounts of financial data securely. It also helps banks serve customer needs to obtain cash and financial data via machine at any time. As hospitals move similarly to expand their scope of service and address the concerns of their stakeholders, they need to have the ability to provide and obtain patient information at any time, direct that information securely to those who have a legitimate need for it, and track patient response to treatment so as to perform quality assurance activities and bill accurately for services rendered.

Currently, some insurers are able to scan every document that is submitted to them as part of the patient record. Thus, invoices, handwritten progress notes, typed reports, and electronically transmitted billing and payment data become easily accessible. For example, the customer service representative or the utilization review nurse can reproduce them on a computer screen. Further, each computer transaction creates an "audit trail" or retrievable log of who processed the claim or handled the customer interaction, increasing the accountability of the insurance representative. As a result, the computer systems also track the productivity of the company employees by measuring how much time they take with each customer, as well as how many claims they "adjudicate" or review and process for payment per hour. This new technology lowers the cost of processing claims and increases the satisfaction of the company stakeholders (e.g., patients, physicians, hospitals, employers).

Electronic Data Interchange. Most efforts to transmit patient data electronically have targeted the billing services. The advancement of electronic data interchange (EDI) and computerization in general promises to transform the business office functions of health care, however. Many clerical jobs in hospitals, physicians' offices, and other settings will disappear because of EDI and computerized transcription of patient records, such as dictated notes from radiology and specialty consults. The skill set to work in the age of EDI will include familiarity with the Internet, e-mail, and the special requirements of payer organizations for accurately coded and transmitted billing and clinical information.

Internet/Intranet. A worldwide network of more than 40,000 interconnected computer networks from more than 70 countries, the Internet comprises academic, government, commercial, and military networks. It functions as a central hub for e-mail and a gateway from one network to another (e.g., sending e-mail from CompuServe to America OnLine). The Internet is a source of information on almost any subject, including medical data and job information.

An intranet, an Internet within an organization, allows personnel to use e-mail, as well as to share data and files. Depending on the network configuration, the system can track individual patients/customers throughout their service encounter. The computer network manager, or the project manager, can monitor each user on the network. The sociologic effect of this technology is that each user becomes a contributor or collaborator in the organization rather than a competitor who holds back ideas and information for personal advantage. Optimally functioning organizations of the future will require free collaboration within the communication structure of the enterprise.

Data Sets

In order for complex systems of health care to work together successfully, it is essential for them to have common definitions of the service constituents (patients), services to be rendered, service elements, and service outcomes. To this end, a number of projects are proceeding to identify data sets within certain areas of health practice.

Data sets are compilations of data elements; each data element (or data point) is a single piece of information. The fundamental data structure in any data-processing system, a data set is defined by size (i.e., characters) and type (e.g., alphanumeric, numeric only, true/false, date) required by an organization. A specific range of values for each data element is also part of the definition.

A number of data sets are currently used in health care. The Health Care Financing Administration (part of the U.S. Department of Health and Human Services) requires collection of the Minimum Data Set (MDS) in Long-Term Care for any patient who stays in a skilled nursing facility for more than 14 days. The Uniform Data Set for Medical Rehabilitation, called the Functional Independence Measures (FIM), measures a patient's functioning on admissions and on discharge to a rehabilitation setting; it also makes it possible to track the diagnosis and financial cost of care. Currently, efforts are under way to identify a minimum data set for home care, hospice, and nursing care. The use of nursing diagnoses to identify a nursing data set creates special problems in that it is difficult to apply nursing diagnoses in the clinical setting.

Nursing diagnosis is couched in language that makes it difficult for other disciplines to understand its usefulness. Phrases such as "the potential for impaired gas exchange" are substituted for "the patient may find it difficult to breathe." The original purpose of the nursing diagnosis approach was to identify a diagnostic approach to discrete issues that nurses face with their patients. The idea was to get nurses on a level with other professionals, such as physicians. However, the practical use of the methodology of nursing diagnoses has not advanced nursing's cause, because, while useful in training, nursing diagnosis does not translate well into day-to-day practice. The

Notes

practical result is that most nursing care plans where nursing diagnosis is mandated are documented in a perfunctory way, then ignored, even by nurses. Further, nursing diagnosis does not benefit patients as well as interdisciplinary care plans that are focused, practical, and progressive. Moreover, because few other disciplines understand it, it is difficult for nurses to communicate with others regarding the judgments they make and the value of their efforts.

CUSTOMER AND PATIENT EXPECTATIONS

Although hospitals have promoted customer service etiquette as the solution to patient dissatisfaction, it is only one perspective. More recent data about patient perceptions indicate that patients feel uninvolved in decisions about their care and feel lost in the health care maze. There is a growing perception that insurance companies are making medical decisions. Patients would like to have their physicians more involved, but the majority of patients who had complaints about the process indicated that they themselves should be in charge of decisions about their care options. There was also some concern that those being discharged after a hospitalization or following outpatient surgery received inadequate explanations. Nearly one-third of patients felt poorly prepared to go home, not knowing the danger signals to watch for, the side effects of their medications, or the time at which they should expect to resume normal activities. Additionally, one-third of the more than 34,000 patients surveyed reported problems getting answers to important questions or talking to caregivers about their concerns.[7]

Patients do not want glossy brochures, smarmy commercials, or even smiling attendants. They want real information about how to get better. They want practical advice available to them as they encounter the day-to-day problems of disease. They want some help navigating the system. They want honest, immediate responses to their concerns. Nurses are often the only practitioners who have the training and are in the right spot at the right time to meet these patient needs. There are many reasons why nurses do not do this. (Some do, but secretly, surreptitiously. To be caught usurping the doctor's prerogative invites confrontation. Many nurses have the knowledge but have a low level of comfort or feel they do not have the time to listen to the patient or to act on patient questions or complaints.)

Many hospital nurses simply do not understand patient care in the home setting. They have not been trained or socialized to think in those terms. For the patient, rehabilitation at home from an acute or chronic illness involves adapting to the illness, having a family caregiver, taking responsibility for self and family, seeking disease-specific practical advice, learning self-care techniques, and developing a willingness to heal and confidence that things will go well. The present system does not yet provide that, although such a service would have a market.

REENGINEERING

The impact of managed care, decreasing levels of reimbursement, declining admissions, and rising expectations by consumers and payers of health care has forced most hospitals to implement efforts to reduce costs and improve the quality of care rendered. Reengineering, as defined by Hammer and Stanton, is "the fundamental rethinking and radical redesign of business process to achieve dramatic improvements in critical, contemporary measures of performance, such as cost, quality, speed and ser-

Notes

vice."[8] Within the hospital setting, reductions in length of stay and resource utilization are the fundamental goals of hospital reengineering efforts, as articulated by Lathrop.[9] The patient-focused care model that Lathrop developed is synonymous with the reengineered hospital. Both terms have many negative connotations among hospital executives and employees alike.

The results of hospital reengineering in the United States are decidedly mixed. Many nurses have indicated that the experience in their institutions was negative. Physicians, middle managers, and lower-level employees tend to be displaced and may not even be consulted about changes in their work.

Reengineering is supposed to redesign business processes radically by reducing the steps involved, the numbers of people required, and the cycle of time needed to complete a process. Changes in job classifications should reflect the broader task responsibilities, and cross-training should be available to help employees function in these expanded jobs. By definition, technology should be assisting with the radically improved processes, either by automating or eliminating labor-intensive tasks. Reengineering should not only reduce cost structures, however; it should also increase revenue and growth. This is a difficult goal in a service industry in which computer and information technology is not yet able to provide information to clinicians at multiple sites so as to improve the efficiency and effectiveness of the medical interventions. Moreover, the information systems are not yet able to provide data concerning the real costs of the interventions in terms of variables such as labor, supplies, and overhead.

Most hospitals that initiate a reengineering program have the reduction of costs as their top priority. Many senior managers recommend reengineering proposals then delegate the tough task of working through the process to team leaders, managers, and department directors. Senior managers should take a proactive stance on reengineering efforts, however, basing their efforts on financial and market projections that include the impact of managed care, briefer hospital lengths of stay, and shrinking Medicare/Medicaid reimbursement.

Benchmarking is one technique used to set goals in reengineering, to identify opportunities for savings, and to spark discussion within work redesign groups. Most benchmarking tends to be financially oriented, partly because reengineering is financially motivated and partly because financial managers are usually charged with measuring the success of the institution's reengineering efforts. Savings are often quantified as directly controllable expenses, labor versus supply expenses, or FTE employee expenses. In general, finance departments define and monitor expense savings and calculations, with an effort to keep the measures uniform within the institution.

Positive results from reengineering processes in the United States generally involve improvements in admission and registration processes, implemention of better case (care) management, and a greater range of the skill mix of personnel in patient care areas. Some departments are combined, such as utilization review and medical records, to increase efficiency.

Missteps and Next Steps

Hospitals have encountered a variety of problems during reengineering efforts. Surveys indicate that the time commitment, especially in the face of the need to continue operations during the reengineering process, is problematic. Finding the money to create additional savings from reengineered processes has been mentioned. Staffing problems are cited, especially on nursing units. Most hospitals anticipate a large increase in training expenses required to fill redesigned job positions.[10]

For many hospitals, it is still too early to tell what the next steps will be in the reengineering efforts. Most are not able to infuse the organization with continued enthusiasm for the process. Few ongoing reengineering projects become part of the everyday culture of the institution. Many hospitals are still in the redesign phase or are just beginning the implementation phase. Some are proceeding through the reengineering process department by department and do not yet have a clear picture of the overall impact of reengineering on the hospital.

Overall, reengineering efforts in health care settings are still in the beginning stages. Most efforts are not comprehensive enough to fit the definition of reengineering. Hospitals have focused largely on reducing costs, not on gaining market share or implementing new programs that provide the organization with strategic advantage. Most efforts focus on tactical issues and incremental improvement, reducing staff without forethought to retraining or retaining. The return on the investment for the reengineering efforts is generally perceived as positive for only a few hospitals.[10,11]

The Nurse's Personal Response to Reengineering

Many nurses have resisted or even sabotaged reengineering efforts in their hospitals. Delaying reengineering only protects the status quo within the organization. The status quo was never that good for nurses, however, and trying to maintain it now will only ensure that the institution will fail to survive in the future.

A more productive tactic is to insist that the reengineering effort be true reengineering, that is, that the focus go beyond cutting costs or downsizing departments. True reengineering addresses the needs of all the customers/stakeholders of the provider organization and then redesigns processes that are more responsive to customer needs, incorporating technology (e.g., computers/information systems), better training, and a renewed sense of organizational mission to help the provider organization service its customers.

CONCLUSION

The modern industrial version of medical care (usually called health care) is disintegrating. It costs more than people and government are able to pay, and it does not address many of the human needs of the people it is supposed to benefit. Changes in the public's perception of the health care system and the impact of technology are forcing radical restructuring. For many health care provider institutions, however, the changes will not ensure their survival in the marketplace. Nurses need to accept the reality that although many of these changes are beyond their control, they may benefit personally from the changes if they can adjust their skill set and view of the world.

NOTES

1. Ernst & Young, LLP, *Health Data Reference Card* (Cleveland, OH: January 1996).
2. Hoechst Marion Roussel, *HMO-PPO Digest* (Kansas City, MO: Hoechst Marion Roussel Managed Care Digest Series, 1996), 16.
3. *The Americans With Disabilities Act, Questions and Answers* (Washington, DC: U.S. Government Printing Office, 1991).
4. Ernst & Young, *Health Data Reference Card.*
5. Ernst & Young, *Health Data Reference Card.*

Notes

6. C. Russell, *What Determines Demand?* (Golden, CO: Health Decisions Inc., 1994).

7. Picker Institute, *Eye on Patients: A Report to the American Public* (Boston: 1996).

8. M. Hammer and S. Stanton, *Reengineering the Corporation: A Manifesto for Business Revolution* (New York: Harper Business Publishers, 1993), 32.

9. P. Lathrop, *Restructuring Health Care* (San Francisco: Jossey-Bass Publishers, 1992).

10. R. Coile and S. Gray, "The Second Wave of Health Care Re-Engineering: New Focus on Processes and Growth," *Health Trends* 9, no. 8 (1994): 1–7.

11. M. Newell, et al., "Reengineering: The New Jersey Experience," *The Garden State Focus* (The Journal of the New Jersey Chapter of the Healthcare Financing Management Association) 43, no. 6 (1997): 5–9.

2

Quality of Care and the Nurse's Role

Nursing has often been viewed as a second-class profession, except in time of war. Therefore, nurses' wages have often been low, and their working conditions have been poor. The nursing shortage of the 1980s resulted from these low wages and poor working conditions, plus the need for more skilled practitioners in the high-technology environment of hospitals. The need for skilled nurses to operate the technology raised wages, and that very technology is continuing to change the role of the hospital. The major employers of nurses have responded to their need to reduce costs by using more nurses in part-time positions and more unlicensed personnel. This has caused a resurgence in union organizing activity in some areas of the country.

NURSES' VIEW

In 1996, the *American Journal of Nursing* conducted a survey of more than 7,000 nurses, the largest survey of nurses' views on health care ever done. Almost 57 percent of the respondents said that the quality of care did not meet their personal standards. In sub-

41

acute care units, only one-third said that they were able to give quality care. Health care providers in the Pacific regions of the United States, where managed care systems are common, were very likely to employ assistive personnel or use part-time employees instead of full-time employees to perform nursing tasks. This led to the perception that continuity of care was significantly decreased within the settings described (i.e., hospitals, subacute and long-term care facilities, and home care). More than 55 percent of nurses, including most geriatric nurses, said they saw more unexpected readmissions of recently discharged patients.[1]

The value or esteem that nurses hold in society will come to the forefront with the aging of the population. More people are living longer than ever before. The number of people who are living past 85 years of age and who require some kind of daily health care intervention is rising twice as fast as the rest of the population. Although most folks have been socialized to view the physician as the arbiter of health, they learn as they age that there are many things that the physician cannot do.

Once patients realize that there is no cure for the chronic conditions brought about by aging or many other components of the human condition, the more realistic patients begin to look for ways to maintain an optimal state of health and functioning (also called health-related quality of life [HRQOL]). Coping with chronic conditions demands practical solutions to everyday problems. Patients and their families need a resource person who knows how the health care system works, what self-care measures can give comfort to a patient, what resources (monetary and otherwise) are available to assist a patient with an evolving disablity, and how a patient and family can meet goals that are important to them. Because nurses can function well in this role, they are the most appropriate kind of health care provider to thrive in the age of managed care.

HISTORICAL VIEW

Although nursing got its start in the household, where women learned to minister to their families, these skills did not grow with the needs of more complex societies. Florence Nightingale codified nursing on battlefields and in the cities of newly industrialized England. She complained that the term *nursing*

> has been limited to signify little more than the administration of medicines and the application of poultices. It ought to signify the proper use of fresh air, light, warmth, cleanliness, quiet, and the proper selection and administration of diet, all at the least expense of vital power to the patient.[2]

Her message was for nurses to have more self-respect and systemization in their nursing practice. Nightingale urged nurses to listen to the voices within them as to how they should proceed in their work.

Nightingale adopted a military (or more correctly, paramilitary) model for her early nursing programs in order to keep order and maintain discipline and training. This helped protect her nurses from the soldiers and gave her some control over the way that the nurses were viewed. The convent-style rules of hospital diploma programs evolved from this approach (along with the fact that nursing was part of the mission for many religious orders), although many hospital programs used the strict discipline to elicit more work from the nursing students than they had a reasonable right to expect.

Physicians' orders were originated by Nightingale as a methodical way to construct a medical record for the patient. They also provided assurance that the physician was performing to an accepted standard and was ultimately responsible for the patient's welfare. Although physicians' orders helped to organize the delivery of care, their use somehow empowered the physician beyond reason. Additionally, the allocation of spatial patterns (the layout of hospitals and clinical care areas) to accommodate physicians has impoverished the nonmedical, health-supporting, and healing aspects of the social and physical environment of modern people.

An easy example of this practice was the advent of critical care units. These care areas evolved from post-anesthesia recovery rooms, where patients came from the operating room to be monitored until their general anesthesia wore off. As patient conditions became more complicated and required close monitoring for greater than several hours, intensive care units (ICUs) evolved. They tended to be near the operating room and were in windowless rooms brightly lit 24 hours a day. There was often no effort on the part of the medical or nursing staff to protect patient privacy or tone down the noise level. Intensive care patients who required mechanical ventilation or other technical support and monitoring were inadvertently subjected to sleep deprivation and other sensory anomalies that led to what we now call "ICU psychosis." Most ICUs have now been redesigned, but the placement of patients in an industrialized environment during the critical phase of their health crisis often leads to unforeseen psychological manifestations.

The shift in women's career choices toward doctoring and lawyering may have contributed to the nursing shortage. Nursing is tied to the traditional, assumed to be women's work, and thus sometimes considered less valuable. Interestingly, Nightingale closed her seminal work *Notes on Nursing* by commenting on the "jargons" or arguments over the proper work of women. She urged every woman to "bring the best she has *whatever* that is, to the work of God's world."[3]

PRESENT VIEW

Nursing's more recent predicament, with the renewed push for low-skilled "nurse-extenders" and the displacement of nurses from the hospital setting, should not be an unexpected action by those who are charged with administering hospitals. After all, nurses are the largest employment group within the institutions. Unless nurses take a cohesive stance, they are easy targets for divide-and-conquer strategies.

Fighting among themselves keeps nurses from addressing the important issues of how resource decisions are made and who has the power to affect nurses' professional practice. It is no secret that hospitals have strived to maintain monopsony control over nursing. Monopsonies are monopolies where a single buyer tries to control the price paid for a product or service offered by many sellers. Hospitals have long attempted to exert control over the wage and working conditions of nurses by communicating with each other regarding wage rates. Nurses have made it easy for others to control their destiny because so many have moved in and out of the labor force, preferring to work when they have the time, eschewing the politics of the workplace, and directing their attention to their families' needs.

Effect of Nursing on Personal Lives

Being a caregiver (and the reasons that they are caregivers) has a big impact on nurses' personal lives. Not only do nurses take care of their patients; they also tend to be the people to whom their family members turn when they have a health problem. Nurses routinely assume the caregiving role—often without thanks. Not being thanked for the thankless jobs tends to devalue the caregiver's contribution and even the caregiver personally, thus distorting the relationship. It is often the nurse, the caregiver in the relationship, who is left responsible for the children, the elderly parents, and so forth. Sometimes, nurses need to take stock and set boundaries about the caregiving burdens that they are willing to assume in the family, both for their own welfare and for the family's welfare. They must take care of themselves in order to take care of others.

Society seems to value those services that are sold on the open market, those which have monetary value. Women throughout the world tend to specialize in nonmarket activities, however, that bring a real sense of quality to their personal, day-to-day lives. Although their work may have lesser market value, it is important for all caregivers to insist on some recognition for the real value of their work. The gift-giving nature of caregiving does have its advantages. Those who are able to care for others tend to have deeper, more meaningful relationships. The altruistic nature of caregiving has positive effects on the caregiver, including a high sense of personal gratification, a feeling of connectedness with others, and evidence of improvement in the functioning of the human immune system.

Ethical Behavior of Caregivers in a Managed Care World

Nursing, as a caregiving profession, is a highly moral enterprise. Most nurses are very aware of their own moral code and avoid morally ambiguous situations. Nurses have seldom been allowed to act as moral agents in hospitals, which may be why so many nurses find more independent practice settings (e.g., home health care) more gratifying.

Clinicians, including nurses, have been socialized to believe that it is not ethical to consider the allocation of resources in reference to patient care. Should it matter that the patient who really needs a service cannot pay for it? The question of resource allocation usually arises even before the patient enters the health center system, however. Many patients who need service but cannot afford to pay for it avoid presenting themselves for care until very (or too) late. Further, will rendering the service ultimately do the patient any good? Will the treatment work if the patient cannot comply with a full treatment regimen? Does rendering treatments that are going to fail constitute ethical behavior?

Perhaps the ethic should be that care is to be rendered only if the patient and family are in a position (i.e., willing and able) to engage in a fully realized treatment plan. If the patient or family cannot comply with the agreed-upon course of treatment (provided that the patient is fully informed about the treatment and its ramifications), perhaps the treatment should be withheld. Then more resources would be available to treat everyone who wished to be treated.

In the age of managed care, the availability of resources is linked to approved treatment plans. Society has seemed to accept this new arrangement as a way to reduce the cost of care. Therefore, nurses are beginning to realize that more efficient and error-free methods of rendering care constitute more ethical forms of caregiving. There is a link between how efficiently nurses give care and how effective that care is. Further, there is a link between the engagement of the patient/family in the treatment plan and the outcome of the treatment. Thus, ethical caregiving behavior has the best chance of succeeding.

CARING VS. CURING

Not long ago, in the days when it was thought that almost every disease had a cure or would soon have a cure, the high-technology acute care focus of modern medicine seemed like a good idea. The basis for this model of disease is a flawed assumption, however—that each disease process (e.g., infection) has a single cause (e.g., exposure to a certain organism). The short-term intervention of technology should be sufficient to "fix" the biology, but nothing is ever that simple in real life. The infection flourishes, proceeding from one person to another because of poor hygiene, inadequate public health (teaching and infrastructure) systems, and the susceptibility of the host organism (human being) to the infection. Further, by using the single weapon of the antibiotic as the major intervention of actual or suspected infections, physicians have inadvertently prompted the mutations of antibiotic-resistant bacteria that cause more virulent infections than the bugs they replace.

The cure model also has problems when applied to broken limbs. Most broken bones, apart from pathologic fractures due to aging or drugs and radiation treatments, happen when the person has been drinking alcohol. The consumption of alcohol triggers many traumatic injuries, such as those that result from motor vehicle accidents. The medical system is unable to address this issue within the model of a cure, because the victims are likely to traumatize themselves or others again under similar circumstances.

Cost of Chronic Conditions

In the 1920s, before the development of antibiotics, health statisticians noted that chronic illnesses were replacing infectious diseases as the predominant health care challenge. By the 1930s, it was noted that although infectious disease was more life threatening, chronic disease was more often disabling. The first national health survey found that 22 percent of the population had a chronic disease, an orthopaedic impairment, or a deficit in vision or hearing. By 1987, 88.5 million noninstitutionalized U.S. citizens, or 46 percent of the population, had one or more chronic conditions; 32 million people had some form of activity limitation due to chronic disease; and 9 million were unable to carry out major activities appropriate to their age. The total direct costs of those conditions accounted for more than 75 percent of all money spent on health care.

Persons with chronic conditions account for 60 percent of hospital admissions and 80 percent of hospital days. Their average length of stay is almost double that of patients who do not have chronic conditions. Almost all of home care use (96 percent), prescription drug use (83 percent), physician visits (66 percent), and emergency department visits (55 percent) are incurred by persons with chronic conditions.[4]

Caring over Curing for Those Who Are Chronically Ill

Most of the people with chronic conditions in the United States are elderly. Within that group, however, only 10 percent of Medicare beneficiaries account for 80 percent of the costs of care. The number of elderly was 37.2 million in 1995, 3.6 million over the age of 85 years. The number of people older than age 65 will grow at the same rate as the general population, or approximately 5 percent per year, although the number of elderly over 85 years of age is growing at an annual rate of 20 percent.

Notes

People who are elderly and chronically ill are looking for the same things that everyone wants: independence, ability to do things that are normal (e.g., have a job and a family, be valued by others). In their struggle for a "normal" human life, they need services to assist them in coping with their condition. The repertoire of interventions to cope with chronic disease includes preventive health care, health education and teaching, practical aspects of overcoming specific limitations or disabilities, and a caring attitude that does not denigrate them or dismiss their view of themselves in the world.

Most baccalaureate nurses have training in general systems theory, giving them a framework for fitting information from other disciplines. Nurses are often required to take on the roles of other disciplines, or to make judgments on the quality or appropriateness of their work. For instance, nurses who do utilization review audits pass judgments on doctors, physical therapists, and other providers; psychiatric nurses perform counseling functions just as social workers, psychologists, or psychiatrists do; and nursing administrators translate program plans that coordinate health programs aimed at addressing the needs of the chronically ill.

With more families faced with caring for a family member who is elderly or has a chronic disease, those who know how to deal with chronic disease and who bring a caring attitude to their work will be more valued as the U.S. population ages. The skill set needed to assist patients who are aging and chronically ill includes those things nurses have always done well: listening, advocating, performing physical assessments, and negotiating resources for patients using their knowledge of the system. Now, in addition, they need to know about physical therapy, counseling techniques, and alternative funding sources for patients. It is up to all nurses and their supporting organizations to position themselves, their training, and their payment mechanisms to take advantage of this emerging opportunity.

With the whole system moving to a corporate model, nurses must find their niche and advocate for themselves and their patients. They must be able to show the value of what they do and not be afraid to ask to be paid fairly to perform these activities. Do they really need multibillion-dollar corporations to hire them and charge a premium for their labor, just because the corporations know how to manipulate the payment system? Is there a better way to do more for patients at lower cost, while still finding a way to make a decent living? This is the challenge for nurses and their professional organizations.

FUTURE OF THE HEALTH CARE BUSINESS

A short time ago, the health care industry was largely a mom and pop enterprise, consisting of many single practitioners (physicians, physical therapists, small community hospitals, locally owned home health agencies and nursing homes). Now hospitals are aligning themselves with each other to carve up regional markets and protect themselves against competition and the managed care organizations. Many local providers of home health care, long-term care, medical equipment, and rehabilitative services are being bought out by large for-profit enterprises. This trend is resulting in the following:

- Many middle management professionals in support services, such as purchasing, human resources, and administrative positions of ancillary departments, are being eliminated. Economies of scale are achievable in larger corporations.
- Larger organizations are investing in technologies to eliminate many other positions, such as

those of clerks who perform transcription and billing services. Voice recognition and document scanning technologies are making these economies possible.

- Weaker hospitals will close. Those communities that depended on their hospital to serve them are bound to be disappointed. Small nonprofit hospitals will not have the economies of scale to compete where larger organizations are in the market. For-profit hospitals are answerable to their board of directors and, apart from goodwill publicity, may give community concerns a low priority.
- Large organizations are beginning to revamp their personnel policies and procedures to be uniform across the entire organization. These policies will conform to higher standards in personnel practice, because the large organization is now at greater risk for lawsuits (partly because the public believes that the organization has "deep pockets").
- Critical paths are being developed and instituted for clinical areas. These paths will assist organizations to collect data on resource utilization and the efficiency of individual physician practices. They will also assist large organizations in managing patients along the entire continuum of care, from the physician's office, to the acute care unit, to the post–acute care settings (e.g., subacute, long-term care), and at home.
- Advances in communications technology will give practices such as telemedicine a boost. Telemedicine includes the viewing of X-ray films, pathology slides, and other data over computer screens from remote areas and will profoundly affect the marketability of some specialists, such as radiologists and pathologists. It will enable better diagnosis and timelier treatments for patients in remote or rural areas.

- The demands of payers and regulators will put more emphasis on the quality of care. These quality data will include patient satisfaction surveys and measurements that focus on the patients' functional health and subjective perception of well-being. These measurements will gradually come into use so that each patient will be surveyed each time he or she seeks care, whatever the setting.
- Though large organizations will strive to have an array of services to meet the needs of most of their service population, many niche opportunities will open up for single practitioners who have expertise with unusual or difficult-to-treat diagnoses. For example, nurses with expertise in wound care who will make home visits can contract with provider organizations who have taken on the risk of all medical needs for a number of patients. In this scenario, the specialty nurse could contribute excellent care and patient satisfaction, while still saving the provider organization money.

Notes

THE FUTURE OF NURSING

In the future, as the patient population gets older, there will be more focus on the caring aspect of health care. However, clinicians, including nurses, will have to operate with computerized equipment that receives the patient record, prompts the appropriate questions, and formats the reports to be forwarded to a central file for viewing by other practitioners who are participating in the patient's care and collecting data for quality purposes.

High Technology vs. Low Technology

Although much fanfare accompanies the use of high-technology health care innovations and interventions, the caring aspect that nurses bring to health care starts with low-technology interventions. The quality of verbal and body language interaction during patient interviews and the quality of the nurse's touch during the examination, for example, still mean a great deal to patients and their outcomes.

Additionally, the intention of the clinician is important. The intention of the practitioner comes through to the patient, and nurses' intentions for patients can have a profound effect on the patients' responses to the interventions. Listening intently while interviewing the patient or while palpating or massaging the body elevates the quality of the encounter for both the patient and the caregiver. (The positive effect of therapeutic touch, which involves no actual touching, is ascribed to the positive, willful intention of the therapist.) High-technology and low-technology interventions are not mutually exclusive. The nurse can combine the quality of low-technology caring with the efficiency of high-technology interventions and communications.

Telemedicine

Long foreseen by the technophiles, telemedicine is now a force to be reckoned with in rural and underserved areas of the world. It is not simply interactive video or picture and telephone conferencing. It can transmit data from electronic stethoscopes, laryngoscopes, and otoscopes. It is useful in radiology, ophthalmology, pathology, dental medicine, and dermatology. It can provide surgical support for unusual procedures when the on-site surgeon needs some expert guidance; it can even allow a faraway expert to "feel" the characteristics of tumors with the assistance of an electronic "glove" communications device. Patients can undergo continuous cardiac monitoring and diagnostic quality electrocardiograms from a remote location,

with and without wires. Pulmonary function tests
and many other procedures can be carried out electronically. All these things can be done with off-the-
shelf equipment that is currently available.[5] Nurse
"physician extender" roles in rural or other hard-to-
serve areas could be advanced by the wide acceptance
of telemedicine. Although most telemedicine advocates see its utility in rural areas, other scenarios are
unfolding. For example, the MercyCare Mobile Health
Program has two vans equipped to perform X-rays,
mammographies, routine lab work, and electrocardiograms and can transmit the data to a central point
for medical record storage and physician interpretation (personal communication with Gloria McNeal,
PhD, RN, CNA, Director, The MercyCare Mobile Health
Program, Landsdowne, PA).

Genetics

The human genome project is now mapping the
whole range of human genes. As this work continues,
more new techniques for using genetic interventions
will unfold. The role of genetic testing in identifying
risks for individuals and populations, and interventions for treating certain kinds of diseases is an area
that will require the counseling and support functions that nurses can provide. Additionally, the ethical issues and research projects that will originate in
this exciting application should open up many opportunities for nurses.

Telephone Support

For patients who are part of a cohesive, coordinated
health care plan, telephone support is taking an in-
creasingly important role. The fee-for-service system

that preceded the rise of managed care had no incentive for providers of care to offer anything more than general education via tele-help lines set up to run prerecorded messages. Now that providers are receiving a fixed, per member (capitated) fee to provide medical and health services for specific populations, telephone support has become a vital service tool.

Telephone support involves sophisticated types of voice-mail that can alert a physician to a patient need, enable monitoring for quality, or transmit information about an emergency that requires a quick response. Quality checks by means of recorded telephone queries prompt subscribers to answer satisfaction surveys and surveys concerning their present health status. Telephone support using nurses varies according to the situations. In some cases, the term "telephone triage" is used when a nurse is called with an acute problem and the patient or family needs to be directed to a specific site for care. More comprehensive programs involve demand management or population management models described below.

Demand Management

A more far-reaching service in which a toll-free number is available to all subscribers is called demand management. Health maintenance organizations (HMOs) have already initiated most of the possible ways to limit the supply of medical services to save themselves money, and they are now turning their attention to decreasing the demand for those services. With demand management, a subscriber may call at any time to obtain advice or health information, to complain about a service, or to seek care. The goals of many demand management companies are to reduce emergency department visits by 60 percent, physician office visits by 50 percent, ambulance services by 60 percent, and overall costs by 25 percent.

Significant reductions in the demand for health services are being made while subscriber satisfaction is increasing.

The idea behind demand management programs is to make health care information freely available so that subscribers can manage their own health care. When unsure or in need of assistance, a subscriber makes a call to a group of highly trained nurses who have access to the subscriber's health record (not yet possible in all demand management programs) and to computer-generated decision support algorithms based on the subscriber's description of the symptoms. Sometimes the subscriber is advised to get to the hospital right away. Sometimes the demand management nurse makes the call and orders the ambulance.

Demand management programs are growing rapidly in use and sophistication. Many train nurses in telephone counseling techniques and are continually updating the algorithms that guide nurses about which questions to ask patients, what further information may be needed, or what direction the patient may be advised to take. Some programs are structured so that any questions that cannot be immediately answered are researched by the nurse and a follow-up telephone appointment is made with the subscriber to discuss the literature search concerning his or her queries. This circumstance may be prompted by rare diseases or unusual patient circumstances.

Demand management programs use the latest information technology support. Some can be used to make referrals for tests or appointments to see a specialist based on the patient's complaint and medical profile. The demand management companies may also compile databases on the lifetime health care needs and physician referrals of each member. This is valuable information in terms of estimating the future costs of care for health care plan members.

Websites/Educational Support

Some large health care insurers, such as US Healthcare, are now planning to use their Website not only as a billboard to show their wares, but also as a tool for subscribers to obtain health information for self-care. Those who want to use such a Website will have to be sanctioned users (i.e., have a subscriber number to gain access). They will also have to know how to do a search using Boolean logic. This system assists in focusing the search by stringing together "keywords" (single words or phrases that can be found in the abstract of a document or in the document itself) with modifiers such as "and," "or," and "not" in a way that focuses the search as tightly as possible.

The term *distributed learning* describes a learning environment that is not a same-time, face-to-face learning environment. Distributed learning is asynchronous, is done over distances, is enabled by technology, and is facilitated by a content expert. It takes advantage of the technology of personal computers with e-mail and groupware (primarily Lotus Notes). This model is perfect for continuing education and adult learners. Each course creates learning teams that, under the instructor's direction, work on group projects and provide a context for the learning experience. Distributed learning is focused and flexible enough for the learning group members to have access to the course materials, assignments, testing materials, and so forth whenever and wherever they wish. Course material can be submitted on specific word processing, spreadsheet, or database programs and sent in packets via e-mail over the World Wide Web to learning (project) team members and then forwarded to the instructor.

Distributed learning software enables group members to learn at their own pace and work on projects that challenge their critical thinking skills. It has the following components:

- schedule database with course syllabus, module assignments, applicable deadlines.
- mediacenter knowledge base and reference tool for course-related content. It can include video clips, computer-based training tools, or graphics.
- courseroom for student discussion between discrete working groups or with the instructor. The instructor usually determines how often the courseroom will be accessed. Courseroom submissions can be graded.
- profiles of students set up like a "homepage" that describes their personal interests and learning objectives.
- assessment manager, an instructor tool for giving evaluations and feedback on student performance, including examinations.

Many learners who may not have done well in a traditional classroom setting do very well with the on-line model. The student who may have been hesitant to give an opinion in front of a live classroom is often willing to take advantage of the relative anonymity of on-line learning to test himself or herself in this type of supportive environment.

The emergence of new models of learning, especially for the adult learner, is an exciting opportunity. Continuing education can proceed in remote areas and at the learner's own pace and schedule.

ALTERNATIVE THERAPIES

Alternative Approaches to Health Bring Opportunities for Nurses

As the present health care system attempts to deal with the challenges of demonstrating value to patients and other customers (insurance companies, governments, unions, etc.), many patients have decided that there is value enough in non-allopathic remedies that they choose to pay out of pocket for these services. Mainstream medicine ignored alternative health care until the publication of the study in the *New England Journal of Medicine* in 1993 that documented that over $10 billion was spent by consumers for alternative health care.[6]

Alternative therapy means different things to different people. As used in the *New England Journal of Medicine* study, *alternative therapy* included chiropractic, a popular drug-free intervention that assists many in coping with maladies that may occur due to mild spinal column injuries. Many chiropractors support a philosophy that encompasses the holistic approach for which alternative medicine is known. Many nurses have gone into chiropractic as a second career.

Alternative medicine generally ascribes to the worldview of holism; that is, that human beings and the world are more than the sum of their parts, that everything is connected. Illness can therefore not be seen out of the context of the person in his or her environment—and that environment is both exterior and interior. Although allopathic medicine has had some success in focusing on disease as an entity, apart from the person, most alternative therapies encompass a systems approach that draws on religious and philosophical tradition. Many people use the terms *wholistic* and *holistic* interchangeably, but there is a difference. "Wholistic" acknowledges the oneness of being in the wider system of people in the world. "Holistic" accepts this, but adds the dimension that the experience of oneness is a peak experience, laden with deep meaning for the individual. Holism gets at the sacredness of peak experiences, the fusion of space and time for the individual. The inducement of holistic experience is often aided by the practice of rituals, as in the practices of aboriginal tribes and other indigenous practices, including shamanism, herbal therapies, faith healing, and incantation prayer ceremonies.

Any nurse who wishes to explore personal or professional opportunities in the field of alternative therapy should expect to fit this into a personal lifestyle that matches the spiritual practices that give alternative healing its extra ingredient of perceived added value to patients and their families. Many people turn to alternative therapies after having failed treatment courses or rejected mainstream approaches. Alternative therapies are still a last resort for most people.

Most successful free-standing holistic health centers have kept their facilities away from the hospitals and avoided conflict with the medical community. Some physicians and other practitioners offer a variety of these services outside of their offices: massage, herbal therapy, nutritional counseling and products, acupressure, yoga, Tai Chi, and so forth.[7]

A number of leading health insurance companies have begun to consider reimbursement for the services of acupuncturists, herbalists, and naturopathic doctors. Oxford Health Plans of New York, Connecticut, and New Jersey is creating a credentialed network of alternative medicine healers who can provide care to those subscribers who have purchased supplemental alternative medicine coverage. Congress is now considering a bill (The Access to Medical Treatment Act) to allow any health practitioner to perform any treatment as long as it is not judged harmful.[8]

Case managers have advocated that patients receive alternative treatments after conventional ones have failed. These "out-of-contract" agreements (called this because the treatments are not stipulated as eligible for payment under the insurance contract) may be approved when there are few viable choices of other therapy, or when the therapy is part of a cultural tradition. Insurance companies need to have a level of comfort with the alternative treatment—they need to know that it will not interfere with any ongoing course of treatment, it will not harm the patient and the ongoing medical treatment, and that the cost and the expected outcome of the therapy are clearly prescribed. Lastly, the therapy proposed for an out-of-contract agreement should be less expensive than treatments normally reimbursed under the insurance contract.[9]

A Systems Approach

A number of exciting theories have emerged that help us understand what a complex system the human body is. Within the space of a generation, mainstream science has moved from the belief that the autonomic nervous system could not intentionally be controlled, to the belief that individuals can learn to control their fight-or-flight response to stress. Visceral learning techniques have been developed that are far more sophisticated than Pavlov's work on salivating dogs. Induced changes in brain chemistry eventually led to the discovery of the role of neuropeptides in the body's response to stimuli. These studies and other sociological studies that looked for a link between stress and the immune system defined the field of psychoneuroimmunology (PNI).

Psychoneuroimmunology

PNI is the study of the brain/nervous system, the immune system, and the hormonal system of the human body as one functioning system. This study has led to advances in the development of some drugs (e.g., serotonin uptake inhibitors, such as Prozac), a better understanding of the role of the brain on emotional experiences and how the body is affected by it, and a better understanding of the chemical receptors for pain and anxiety.

The brain and nervous system were once thought to be like a giant electrical switching system. Add to that the idea of the immune system commanding the body to make judgments differentiating self from non-self. If the immune system fails at a cellular level, the body is exposed to death. But the immune system may mismatch judgments or learn confused and maladaptive messages under stress. The hormonal system enables the brain to respond to the flood of neuropeptides and their receptors to affect feeling states, mental and conscious thinking states, and human behavior. The newly realized brain, as defined by PNI, has placed people at the threshold of new discoveries about the brain, health, and human behavior.

Robert Ornstein's work[10] examines the complex interaction between the brain and environment. The brain's role is to control the internal environment of the body and to maintain homeostasis. The brain screens information, simplifies judgments, stores memory, and compares salient aspects of events to assist people in making judgments. All these functions occur simultaneously and below the conscious level. Conscious, objective reality is a mental caricature, causing many errors in judgment, and some of the behaviors that emanate from these errors become engrained in our subconscious. These patterns of thought may be repeated over generations. Ornstein believes that one of the aspects of human stress is that, for so much of human existence, everything needed to be thought of as a threat. Humans have been living in secure shelter without having to worry about predators for a very short historical time. It is now evident that the fight-or-flight mechanism that was so essential during primitive times is now an inappropriate and maladaptive response to the stresses of modern human existence. This continuing stress shortens lives and impairs the quality of life. A cultural evolution needs to happen for humans to be able to adapt to stress in a more effective way. This evolutionary process can be accelerated by changes in the ways health care is conceived and delivered. In particular, holistic approaches will have a profound effect on this development.

How Patients Present Their Needs

Mainstream medicine's biggest failing is the continued focus on finding a cure, even when there is no cure possible. In fact, most visits to doctors are not caused by disease but are due to complaints of illness that are somaticized. Somaticizers are people whose medical problems are actually physical manifestations of emotional conflicts that remain unconscious. These patients account for 60 to 70 percent of physician office visits and routinely have medical costs 10 to 14 times higher than the national average.[11]

These data show that many patients experience uncontrolled stress in their internal environment. This is true for all patients, including those with legitimate medical conditions. From a nurses' point of view, any approach to support the patient in a way that enables his or her natural healing abilities to respond to stress would fit nursing and holistic therapy. From this point of view, holistic nursing could be practiced in almost any setting, because the nurse could bring (and most *do* bring) a special quality to their relationships with many patients. Nurses are often able to engage patients as human beings and respond to their needs.

Experienced nurses have a repertoire of methods to help patients feel better. These interventions may be of a practical or medical nature, or may involve

comfort measures or psychological and spiritual measures, both for the patient and the family. Holistic
practice is gained from years of experience and the
challenge of patients' health needs.

Historically, nursing has emphasized the art of
healing rather than the need for a cure. The practice
of nursing tends to be altruistic, connected with
feelings for patients, and guided by practical reason-
ing rather than theoretical adherence to narrowly
defined treatment regimens.

Focus on Healing

One aspect of the overwhelming human experience of being sick is the characteristic feeling of
aloneness. This aloneness disconnects one from others, often both physically and emotionally. On the
other hand, healing is an experience of oneness with
others and feeling connected and purposeful. The
holistic approach is essential for a practice that recognizes the healing aspect over the goal of a cure. The
cure is just one dimension of healing. Other dimensions are emotional or psychological, transpersonal
or spiritual, interpersonal or global, in the sense that
we feel connected to others that face the same destiny
and must face the same hurdles in life.[12]

Healing is about allowing the person's natural recovery to take place by supporting him or her through
crises. It also employs the practice of directed intentionality or prayer.[13] Intentionality is an important
component of all hands-on interventions. Patients
can feel the difference when the physical caring is
done with good intent. It makes them feel cared for at
a time when they are most vulnerable and most in
need of feeling connected to others. Healing is the
realization of oneness.[14]

Notes

Matching Holistic Health and Human Behavior

Practitioners may feel that a health intervention has value, but that value needs to be demonstrated to patients and payers. Holistic health interventions allow people to incorporate self-care, stress reduction, and spiritual practices into their everyday life. In this way, holistic health elevates the everyday experience to another level, incorporating a sense of the sacred into how human beings treat themselves, their bodies, and each other.

Eastern religions and philosophies have been a guide to Westerners in this regard. For example, Taoism has been a rich source of inspiration to Western philosophical thought and to other Eastern religions including Buddhism and Hinduism.

Taoist Practice Focuses on Breath and Energy

The Tao (Way or Path) is a central principle that acknowledges the life force in the universe (or Chi). The symbol of the Tai Chi (Figure 2–1) represents the Taoist core belief: dichotomies of opposites make up the universe. These opposite forces (the yin and the yang) interact with each other; the opposites are heaven and earth, light and shadow, warmth and cold, motion and stillness. When there is balance, the result is harmony and good health. However, the yin-yang symbol and the commentaries regarding the symbol were written in primitive times in a patriarchal society. Many positive characteristics are assigned to the male yang, and negatively connoted characteristics to the female yin; but the Tao describes the wise man as one who has many female attributes. Lao Tsu's *Tao Te Ching* (The Way of Life) described the

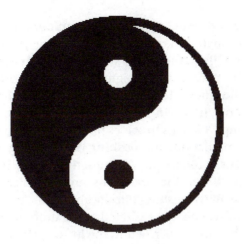

Figure 2–1 Symbol of Tai Chi

Way as a mother, and the ideal realm is described as female.[15]

The symbol of the Tai Chi represents movement. It is sometimes called the "symbol of the two fishes" because it appears as though two fish are chasing each other's tail. The flow of energy generated by the interaction of these opposites is said to be the origin of life energy. The practice of Chi-Kung (breathing exercises), Tai Chi (movement meditation and martial arts exercise), and various other meditation exercises utilizing sounds, stretching, and ritualized movements make up the core of Taoist practice.[16]

The practice of Tai Chi strives for disengagement of confusing or distracting physical surroundings so that cleansing of the internal body can take place. The practice starts with the energizing Chi-Kung breathing exercises. The power of the Tai Chi practice is actualized by moving the energy/breath around the body and concentrating it in different parts of the body. For example, one of the first exercises is the "Microcosmic Orbit" where the breath is brought into the body and moved along the midline axis of the body through chakras, or centers of energy, that transform and distribute it as it streams through them.

Breath energy may be heightened by different breathing techniques. The Chinese claim that prebirth, or embryonic, breathing is one of the most effective for capturing Chi. This involves pulling the abdomen in during inhalation, and pushing it out during exhalation. This is analogous to the fetus, which received nutrients from the umbilicus and expelled or returned flow by pushing out the abdomen. The practitioner moves energy gathered at the umbilicus along a meridian to the perineum, the lower back, the mid-thoracic area, the base of the neck, the top of the head, to a point between the eyes, under the nose, to the lower lip, to the trachea, to the heart, and back to the umbilicus. The Chinese ascribe many illnesses to energy getting stuck at one point or another, or to the buildup of heat due to blocked energy flow within organs in the body. The meditational breathing practices of Chi-Kung and movement practice of Tai Chi are designed to assist the flow of energy and breath.

Other Eastern religious and philosophical traditions often focus on breath and energy flow as a source of healing. The practice of Hinduism describes the Kundalini, or snake, as a sleeping spiritual force that lies at the base of the spine. Through yoga breathing exercises it arises through the chakras to find expression in the form of spiritual knowledge and mystical visions. The energy itself is said to arise in a wavelike pattern, like a snake. Yogic and tantric practices also use many two-syllable formulas, or mantras, that symbolize ongoing inhalation and exhalation.[17]

Craniosacral Therapy

More modern healing practices also take the idea of breath and energy into account when treating injury and illness. The practice of craniosacral healing origi-

nated with an osteopath and is based on the rhythmic movement of the central nervous system. The brain itself expands and contracts, the cerebrospinal fluid moves in waves as it bathes the brain and spinal column, the membranes covering the brain and spinal cord are in motion, and the skull and sacrum have rhythmic motions. Craniosacral therapy involves bringing the skull and spinal cord back into alignment so that the natural rhythmic movement of the structures can resume naturally.[18]

Thought Field Therapy

Another interesting therapy that recognizes the movement of energy waves through the body is Thought Field Therapy™ (TFT). Developed by a psychologist, Robert Callahan, PhD, TFT is the study of thought fields and the body's energy system as they pertain to the diagnosis and treatment of psychological problems. This therapy consists of inducing the negative feeling that characterizes the problem and finding where the energy flow is being blocked along the body's meridians, tapping the body's meridians in a specific order while the patient is concentrating on the psychological problem that causes the disturbance. The meridians are the same ones that acupuncture or acupressure therapists use during their treatments, with the similar intention of freeing the flow of energy throughout the body. Training in TFT has three tiers and minimally involves learning the 14 treatment points and numerous algorithms designating location and sequence of body tapping and energy balancing. Detection and treatment of blocks to successful treatment, called psychological reversal, are an integral part of the success of this therapy. TFT reports an 80 to 90 percent cure rate as brief therapy

Notes

for phobias, addictive urges, and post-traumatic stress disorder.[19]

Conclusion

Changing behavior through holistic therapies that are nontoxic alternatives to the technologic instruments of medical practice is the next great challenge for health practitioners. The purpose of these therapies should be to induce changes in feeling states, resulting in changes in behavior. Positive results may help patients and clients to change their behavior and further adapt to healthier living habits. These habits need to be anchored in belief systems that are harmonious with each individual's life. It is hoped that patients will develop a lifestyle that enhances their quality of life, whether they are faced with chronic illness or the everyday stress and strains of modern living.

ROLE OF THE PATIENT AND FAMILY

The development of managed care, along with high-speed communications, is changing the role of the patient and the family. The physician and the hospital were at the center of the health care universe in the past, but the patient and the family should be at the center of the emerging model. The patient and the family should be seen as a single unit, with similar, but not always agreed upon goals, similar culture and values, and a support system to be optimized for the good of the family as a whole. Patients and families should be viewed as a single unit because most of their values, behaviors, and beliefs are developed in their family life. The family will likely function as the primary caregiver to the patient and will need to understand the patient's medical status and the ramifications of the treatment to support the patient through the rigors of the treatment regimen. Often, issues regarding noncompliance can be successfully addressed if the family is included in the treatment decision making along with the patient.

Current limitations on the availability of health resources mandate that each family learn how to be more self-reliant and how to lower risks against disease. Stress reduction, lifestyle modification, self-awareness, and a moderate exercise regimen can help family members to maintain a high level of health-related quality of life even as they age.

Close family support is not all that is needed in the face of debilitating disease or catastrophic illness or injury. Research shows that the circle of support outside the family can be a very effective factor in recovery. Friends, church members, and neighbors can have a profound effect on the ability of a patient and family to cope with disease.

CONCLUSION

Nurses who are going to survive personally and professionally in the future will survive a trial by fire that clarifies the role of the caregiver and nurse in the postindustrial society. This new vision must accompany a renewed sense of the value of what nurses do: caring, coaching, counseling, educating, and continuing to learn more about the process of healing. Although the tools to accomplish these goals must include high-technology components as they become available, the low-technology aspects of teaching, touch, and intentionality will still be the most value-added activities that nursing has to offer.

NOTES

1. J. Shindul-Rothschild et al., "Where Have All the Nurses Gone?" *American Journal of Nursing* 96, no. 11 (1996): 25–39.

Notes

2. F. Nightingale, *Notes on Nursing* (London: Harrison, 1859), 6.

3. Nightingale, *Notes on Nursing*, 76.

4. C. Hoffman et al., "Persons with Chronic Conditions: Their Prevalence and Costs," *JAMA* 276, no. 18 (1996): 1473–1479.

5. *Telemedicine Today*, 1997 Buyer's Guide and Directory (Shawnee Mission, KS).

6. R. Eisenbert et al., "Unconventional Medicine in the United States," *New England Journal of Medicine* 328, no. 7 (1993): 246–252.

7. J. Shuster, "Wholistic Care: Healing a Sick System," *Nursing Management* 28, no. 8 (1997): 56–59.

8. R.M. Henig, "Medicine's New Age," *Civilization* 4, no. 2 (1997): 42–49.

9. M. Newell, *Using Case Management to Improve Health Outcomes* (Gaithersburg, MD: Aspen Publishers, 1996), 86.

10. R. Ornstein, *Multimind* (Boston: Houghten Mifflin, 1986) and R. Orstein and P. Erlich, *New World, New Mind* (New York: Doubleday, 1989).

11. C. Cummings, "Somatization: When Physical Symptoms Have No Medical Cause," in *Mind–Body Medicine*, ed. D. Goleman and J. Gurin (Yonkers, NY: Consumer Report Books, 1993), 221–232.

12. J. Achterberg, *Woman as Healer* (Boston: Shambhala Publications, 1990).

13. Shuster, "Wholistic Care," 57.

14. J.S. Goldsmith, *Realization of Oneness: The Practice of Spiritual Healing* (Secaucus, NJ: The Citadel Press, 1974).

15. L. Tsu, *Tao Te Ching: A New Translation*, trans. by R.B. Blakney (New York: Times Mirror Publishers, 1955).

16. T.H. Jou, *The Tao of Tai-Chi Chuan: Way to Rejuvenation* (Warwick, NY: The Tai Chi Foundation, 1981).

17. J. Huang and M. Wurmbrand, trans., vol. I and II, *The Primordial Breath* (Torrance, CA: Original Books, 1987).

18. A. Weil, *Spontaneous Healing* (New York: Alfred A. Knopf Publishers, 1995), 25–39.

19. R.J. Callahan, A Thought Field Therapy Algorithm for Trauma: A Reproducible Experiment in Psychotherapy (Paper delivered at the annual meeting of the American Psychological Association, New York, August 1995).

3

Value Added in Nursing Practice

The term *value-added* is a consultant's code word indicating that the high price paid for the services he or she provides is worth the money. Products that are value-added stand out because the customer clearly sees the advantage of the service and is willing to pay the price. Some products and services defy the law of supply and demand because no one knows how to judge their value. Health care is one of the services that falls into this category. Health care defies the normal concept of value in a number of ways. Because it is a service whose outcome cannot be guaranteed (or sometimes even predicted), its quality is difficult to measure. Further, medical care is steeped in mystery for most consumers; they are not the direct payer in most instances, and they have no idea how to judge the value of health care.

VALUE IN HEALTH CARE DEFINED

For many years, physicians held themselves up as the arbiters of quality care. They lost their credibility in setting the price of care, however, when the public, employers, and the government (the payers) noted that the cost of care was increasing, but the quality was not. Managed care companies have shown that their system of prepaid care is at least no worse, and is sometimes better, than fee-for-service physician care.

Certainly, everyone would like someone to define the quality, the value, of the health care and medical services rendered. People would be able to shop for health services as they shop for potato chips. The supermarket shelf has an array of products with the weight, the ingredients, the unit price, and the price per pound clearly marked. Buyers know what they are getting when they buy potato chips. In contrast, when they buy health services, they really do not know what they are buying. They often are not even informed of the price beforehand.

Value is a function of utility over price. Utility, the usefulness of the service, is best defined by the customer, not the provider of services. In regard to health services, the customer's ability to function in a role that he or she considers normal is the ultimate measure of value. People who are unable to function in their normal role—a husband or wife, a caregiver for their family, a breadwinner, a contributor to their community of friends and interests—hold that their life has less value.

Does the person who pays a high price for services get a better value? If the answer to that question is not clear, the value is questionable. The continuing price escalation for health care insurance and health care services begs for continued innovation and redefinition of the concept of value, as well as our concept of health. Defining our value in the health care arena and the value of our life's work, then, is a function of our value system. What are those events and feelings that are most important to us?

Comfort Zone

One great way for people to define their values is to explore their comfort zones. Whom do they like to be with, and what do they like to be doing? What can they do well, and what do they dream of doing if they had the freedom to dispense with the realities of day-to-day living?

Conversely, what do they not like to do? Whom do they not like to be with? Often, circumstances force nurses to work with people and in situations that they would not choose. They need to define more clearly their level of comfort with each aspect of their life to define their values. They also need to let their values and their discomfort motivate them to change their situation.

Personal Goals

Comfort levels and dreams can lead nurses to define their goals. These goals need not always be goals of accomplishment or of acquisition of material goods. They can be goals of feelings or perceptions of self in terms of what they would like to become and how they would like others to perceive them. These are goals of meaning, goals that put our life in a context.

People define the meaning in their lives based on their personal stories; the stories that they narrate about themselves as they try to make sense of their experiences in the world. The narration takes place in their mind, with their own inner voices telling them how to interpret events and how to respond to people. The narration of their life stories is inseparable from their self-perception. People should be comfortable with listening to their voice and should let it guide them, rather than doing things that contradict their inner self. Many people do what they think other people want. If the goals are not genuinely their own, however, people cannot truly find the right goals, lifestyle, or methods of achieving their goals.

HEALTH DEFINED

In his definition of stress, as described in his discussion of the general adaptation syndrome, Selye posited that the body strives to maintain a balance between the inner and outer environment. He called this concept "heterostasis."[1] Health is a relative state of balance and comfort between these environments. The outer environment can include such aspects as the physical environment of the weather, the body's ability to adapt to the weather, the stresses of the work-a-day world, noise, and noxious stimuli.

The general adaptation syndrome has three phases:

1. alarm, where the body reacts to the stressor and produces tension (fight/flight)
2. resistance, where the body tries to cope with the stress by increasing the body metabolism (an inflammatory reaction)
3. exhaustion, occurring after the stressful period has passed or the body can no longer cope with the continued stress

A visualization of the general adaptation syndrome is shown in Figure 3–1.

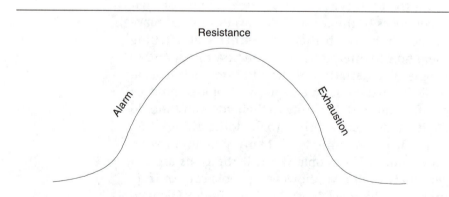

Figure 3–1 General adaptation syndrome

Continuous stress and the body's reaction to it have serious consequences. One result may be hypertension, which is a key component of the number 1 and number 3 causes of death in the United States: heart attack and stroke, respectively.[2] The ability to handle the "noise" of the environment, the unpatterned stimuli that provoke the stress reaction; to block out unwanted noise/stress; and to recognize patterns of stimuli and take advantage of the lessons those patterns teach largely determines a person's success in turning the stimulus of stress into a positive experience.

Figure 3–2 illustrates a series of waveforms that can be seen on any monitor in any intensive care unit (ICU). They measure the amplitude of the pressure inside the pulmonary artery, the arterial blood pressure, and the intercranial pressure. Critical care physicians and nurses work hard to measure and manipulate the frequency and the amplitude of these waveforms accurately so as to increase their patient's chance of survival. Very slight differences in the pressures that the waveforms represent (as little as the weight of several cubic centimeters of water) can mean the difference between life and death for a critically ill patient. The success of critical care medicine and nursing depends on achieving a balance of pressures, a balance between the assaults on the body and the body's ability to cope with the stress.

In order to cope with the stress of life, people must have a sense or belief that they will be able to do so

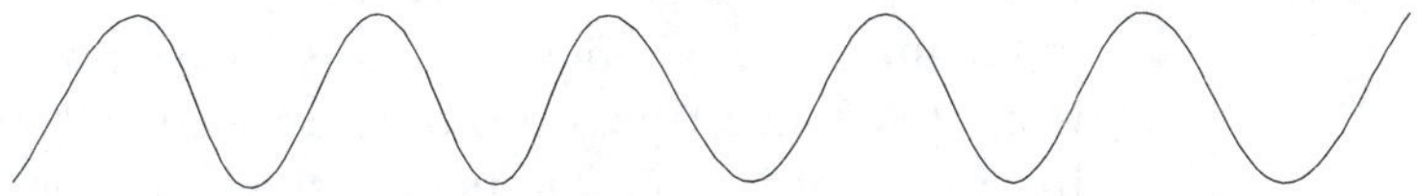

Figure 3–2 Series of waveforms

Notes

successfully. Their appraisal of themselves in their environment will determine how strongly they will work to adapt and change. Their belief that they can influence their own experience, their sense of commitment or involvement in the process, and their sense of challenge that the problem is an opportunity rather than a threat are important arbiters of coherence. Health, then, is contingent on a person's appraisal of his or her ability to cope successfully with "the slings and arrows of outrageous fortune."[3]

As good health is one of the functions of the quality of our lives, so is personal success. The waves that bring us up and down as we live our everyday life are not dissimilar to the waveforms illustrated in Figure 3–2. Success can be measured in a number of ways: the gaining of one's sea legs, the navigation of currents in our personal or professional life, or survival without drowning. Successes can also be a function of whether we are able to anticipate the wave and ride its crest to achieve personal success.

CORPORATE VALUE

Corporations are run by people who measure value in numbers: dollar figures, ratios of dollars earned in relation to industry norms, earnings per share of stock. The decision makers (e.g., the chief financial officer, the comptroller) have financial backgrounds. Nothing is purchased, no project blessed until they approve the cost and the potential for return to the company.

More progressive companies try to infuse their employees with values that are congruent with teamwork, maximum efficiency, and customer satisfaction. They also try to promote a sense of "strategic intent," that is, an awareness of the short-term goals of the company that every employee should know so as to increase the sense of teamwork.

Value of Health Care Services

In the health care field, the emerging companies are forging new identities based on traditional values: caring, excellence, attention to detail. Past success in health care came from maximizing profits by maximizing utilization of services. Hospitals and most other health providers have done this all the while not knowing their true cost of delivering care. Now that hospitals and other health care providers have to learn to be more efficient to ensure that they make money under fixed payment or capitated systems, they do not have enough information about their costs to begin to change the way in which they deliver clinical care.

One way to begin to manage costs is to identify those patients and physicians who incur the highest costs. Using the so-called Pareto principle as a rule of thumb, managers focus on the 10 to 20 percent of patients who account for 80 to 90 percent of the costs of care.[4] Figure 3–3 is an illustration of the bell curve in which where there is a mean (average) cost per diagnosed patient. One standard deviation above and below the mean typically accounts for 68 percent of the patients. Care for the top 16 percent (above one standard deviation) tends to cost less than the average; care for the bottom 16 percent tends to cost more. Therefore, the health care provider that can correctly identify high-cost patients at the start of the encounter can more effectively manage the costs of these patients, even though they may not yet have the controls in place to measure exactly what it costs to provide a unit of care.

In the future, many organizations will be able to track their costs per unit of service by using improved information systems and linking time and resources to diagnostic categories. For the time being, however, many organizations can benefit from a comprehen-

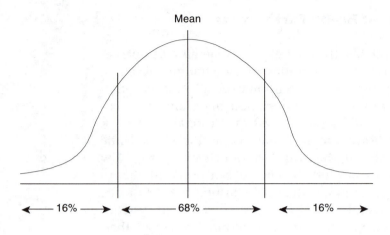

Figure 3–3 Bell curve

sive screening process to identify patients who—because of depression, poor self-rated health, poor family support system, or some other factor—may not respond to conventional treatments rendered in the typical medical care setting. Nurses' ability to identify these patients and adjust the treatment plan to focus on reasonable patient-defined outcomes allows them to bring an added level of value to their organization and to the most problematic patients.

For example, George is a 78-year-old man brought to the hospital for cardiac chest pain. Although he did not have a heart attack, his age and symptoms suggest coronary artery disease. His cardiologist recommends a cardiac catherization and suggests the need for possible surgery. Because the hospital has a risk contract mandating that it pay for all the health services George may require, George is seen by a nurse case manager. The case manager has a series of questions for George as part of her assessment including a health status questionnaire and a health risk appraisal. It becomes clear that George has not been feeling well for some time and he has been living alone since his wife died one year ago. He expresses his fear of the suggested operation and his doubt that it will help him regain an increased level of activity, similar to what he had when his wife was still alive. George also appears depressed and admits to problems sleeping.

If George is depressed, does not think the operation will benefit him, does not have anyone to care for him after the operation, and does not feel that the operation will improve his quality of life, then proceeding with the operation in the face of this evidence is ill-advised. An alternative treatment plan that would address George's depression and lack of family support, and include a trial of medication to address his cardiac condition would be a much more appropriate and cost-effective approach.

Value of Nursing Services

If the level of service provided by a nurse shows that the nurse is personally involved with a patient's real problems, that patient is much more aware of the value of the service. Therefore, if nurses want to be able to show value, in whatever setting they work, they need to find a way to spend more quality time at the bedside.

There are a number of ways to do this. Nurses who are employed by a large organization can volunteer for one of the reengineering teams so that they can influence the inevitable restructuring. In the process, the nurses can build relationships with other members of the reengineering team to gain some insight into the way in which changes will be made, to practice working in the group setting, and help to ensure a job in the future.

Nurses can also look for opportunities to participate in areas such as the development of clinical paths,

Notes

quality improvement, risk management, and utilization management so as to learn more about these important areas and try out new ways to view the practice of nursing. The bottom line for patients (because the customer is the final arbiter of quality) is their perception of the care that they receive. Anything that the nurses can do to make the patients feel that their needs are addressed will benefit the health care organization. This area of endeavor requires a skill set important for any nurse who wants to build a career and be part of a successful organization.

PUBLIC PERCEPTIONS OF VALUE

Often, the perception of value by the public has little to do with reality. Because of the power of advertising, for example, many people are convinced (not rationally, but through associations repeated in all types of media) that drinking a cola will make them feel better. Not only will it make them feel better, but the act of drinking the cola has intrinsic value. It shows that they are discriminating consumers. The essence of advertising is to convince the consumer that there is value in the product that is not inherent to the product. That is, sell the sizzle, not the steak.

To enhance patients' perception of the value of their services, therefore, nurses must convince patients that they get something extra from those services, whether as a group or individually. Identifying that something extra requires some market research with patients and employers. Nurses should ask each patient directly what he or she expects from them. Asking patients directly can clarify their perceptions and make it possible for nurses to adjust their efforts in order to address patient needs more specifically. Those nurses and those organizations that intend to

survive the changes in health care services must become more attuned to the patient's expectations.
They also need to be attuned to the expectations of all
the other customers of their service (e.g., the insurance company, the family, the referral sources).

CONCLUSION

As an industry, health care providers need to reas-
sess their personal attitudes and behaviors with respect to their treatment of customers. Nurses need to
find out more about what patients want, how they
think, and what their perception of the value of
nursing is. Nurses also need to examine their individual skill sets to ensure that there is a place for them
in the health care system of the future.

NOTES

1. H. Selye, *Stress without Distress* (New York: J.B. Lippincott, 1974).
2. J.B. McKinlay and S.M. McKinlay, "A Review of the Evidence Concerning the Impact of Medical Intervention on Recent Mortality and Morbidity in the United States," *International Journal of Health Services* 19 (1989): 181–208.
3. W. Shakespeare, *Hamlet, Prince of Denmark*, Act II, Scene 2.
4. R.J. Coffey and E.J. Gaucher, *Total Quality in Healthcare* (San Francisco: Jossey-Bass Publishers, 1993), 388–389.

4

Identifying the Skill Set for Success

A "skill set" is an individual's group of abilities. If that individual is a nurse, these skills need to match the proficiencies demanded by the nursing practice setting if the nurse is going to be successful. The organization may need to train those who lack the skills but have the aptitude for the kinds of activities needed. For example, certain individuals are more easily trained in the use of laptop computers than others. Those who can adapt to the skills required in changing settings should be of particular value to the organization.

In an analysis of the types of work that people do, Reich described three basic kinds of work: (1) routine production, such as manufacturing or clerical work; (2) in-person service, such as retail or restaurant work; and (3) symbolic analysis.[1] Most people view nursing as a combination of the first two types of work in that nurses perform processes involving the production of paperwork and give hands-on service to people through the technical processes identified with patient care (e.g., passing medication, setting up equipment). Approximately 90 percent of all work involves these first two types.

Symbolic analysts make up the remainder of the work force. Their work involves solving problems,

85

taking lessons learned from one setting and applying them to another, and negotiating or brokering services and fees on behalf of clients. They earn more money than routine production workers or in-person servers because their work is perceived to have greater value. Chief executive officers of large corporations, actuaries, stockbrokers, scientists, and successful artists (e.g., filmmakers, novelists) can demand a premium for their work.

Symbolic analysts not only are adept at systems thinking, but also have a number of skill sets, both technical and social. They need to be able to collaborate with diverse groups of people and guide projects toward a goal. They need to bring a repertoire of techniques to the problem-solving process. They have the capacity to find out what works and what does not work, as well as a willingness to experiment with new ways to solve problems. They can critically analyze the proposed solutions.

IDENTIFICATION OF TRANSFERABLE SKILLS

Because symbolic analysts make the most money in this society and because nurses do many of the same things, nurses should examine their skills to discover what they can do that fits this high-value category.

Exhibit 4–1 is a work history worksheet. It provides for a listing of all positions, paid and unpaid. It is useful to make an expansive list of job duties, responsibilities, and things done well. The last column, which addresses things not liked or not done well, should help rule out future positions with the same requirements.

Exhibit 4–2 focuses on technical proficiencies and people skills acquired through both formal and informal education, including self-improvement activities. This worksheet should be filled out with a com-

Exhibit 4-1 Transferable Skills Worksheet for Nurses: Work History

Start/Stop Dates of Work (Enter Most Recent Job First)	Name of Organization/ Dept.	Description of All Duties or Activities	Responsibilities of Job, Fully or Partially (Be Expansive)	Successes: Things You Did Well and Enjoyed Doing	Limitations: Things You Did Not Do Well/Did Not Like

Exhibit 4-2 Transferable Skills Worksheet for Nurses: Educational Achievements (Formal and Informal Education, Including Self-Improvement)

Date/Setting for Schooling or Training	Area of Concentration	Subject of Projects, Articles, Presentations	Obstacles Encountered	Abilities or Skills Utilized in Overcoming Obstacles	Special Proficiencies Acquired, Including Technical and People Skills

pleted Exhibit 4–1 worksheet at hand so that no on-the-job training or skills learned informally at the workplace are overlooked. Technical and social skills practiced, even if there is no sense of proficiency, should be listed at this point.

Exhibit 4–3 lists credentials and goals achieved as recognized by others. People often forget or disregard recognition or credentials received in past years or in settings different from their present work life. Reviewing these credentials and skills can trigger a different perspective and sometimes a renewed sense of self-confidence, however.

Exhibit 4–4 is to be filled out after each of the other worksheets is completed and at hand. Skills learned and recognized, and obstacles overcome, should be listed in order of their importance. After the priority listing is made for the first column, each skill or ability is broken down into the subskills required to gain proficiency in that skill. Similar or like talents, skills, and activities enjoyed are then analyzed and rephrased in terms of the skills used by highly paid professionals: problem identification and solution; information finding and information systems (e.g., computer and computer search skills); and negotiating skills with people, including coaching and counseling skills.

NURSING SKILL SET MATRIX

Nurses can use an additional worksheet (Exhibit 4–5) to assist them in sorting out their particular skills and identifying the settings in the nursing job market that may require those skills. They simply check off their skills in the column of boxes that lies under the place where they work or would like to work to determine whether they have the appropriate skills for the identified setting. If they sense that they have

Exhibit 4–3 Transferable Skills Worksheet for Nurses: Formal Credentials

Credential or Special Recognition Received	Date Received/ from Whom	Performance Required or Achievement Needed To Gain Recognition	Obstacles Overcome in the Course of Reaching Goal	Abilities Utilized To Overcome Obstacles	Proficiencies Demonstrated for Each Credential or Recognition

Exhibit 4–4 Transferable Skills Worksheet for Nurses: Transferable Skills Analysis

Enter Name or Description of Skills Identified in Previous Worksheets	Specify the Subskills in Each Skill Entered in First Column. What Talents Are Evident?	Rephrase Skills and Talents in Terms of Activities Performed by Symbolic Analysts: (1) Problem Identification/Solving, (2) Information Finding/Systems, and (3) Negotiating/Coaching

Exhibit 4–5 Nursing Skill Set Matrix

	Acute Care	Subacute Care	Long-Term Care	Home Hth[1]	Behv Hth[2]	Dis Mgt	Dem Mgt	Qual Mgt[3]	CM[4]	Alt Hth[5]	UM[6]
Reading/understanding of technical instructions											
Complex calculations of											
Health statistical data											
Financial data											
Personal computer skills											
Word processing											
Spreadsheet											
E-mail											
Internet search											
Database manipulation											

continues

Exhibit 4–5 continued

	Acute Care	Subacute Care	Long-Term Care	Home Hth[1]	Behv Hth[2]	Dis Mgt	Dem Mgt	Qual Mgt[3]	CM[4]	Alt Hth[5]	UM[6]
Presentation graphics											
Fine motor skills											
Insertion of intra-venous lines											
Physical examination											
Set up and trouble-shooting of clinical computer equipment (e.g., monitoring devices)											
Physical skills											
Bending, lifting, stooping											
Working evening/ night shifts											
Tolerating noxious sights/smells											

continues

Exhibit 4–5 continued

	Acute Care	Subacute Care	Long-Term Care	Home Hth[1]	Behv Hth[2]	Dis Mgt	Dem Mgt	Qual Mgt[3]	CM[4]	Alt Hth[5]	UM[6]
Telephone skills											
Telephone repartee											
Pleasant telephone voice and manner											
Writing skills											
Business reports											
Policy/procedures											
Sales letters											
Clear directives											
Academic reporting											
Presentation skills											
Public speaking											
Jokes											
Computer graphics											
Critical thinking skills											
Organizational skills											
Listening skills											

continues

Exhibit 4-5 continued

	Acute Care	Subacute Care	Long-Term Care	Home Hth[1]	Behv Hth[2]	Dis Mgt	Dem Mgt	Qual Mgt[3]	CM[4]	Alt Hth[5]	UM[6]
Negotiating skills											
Counseling skills											
Personality type sets											
Relater											
Socializer											
Thinker											
Doer											

[1]Home health
- Medicare certified
- intravenous care
- wound care
- ventilator care
- high-risk newborn
- newborn
- geriatric
- HIV+/AIDS

[2]Behavioral health
- drug abuse
- alcohol abuse
- sexual addictions
- schizophrenia
- depressive disorders
- psychological counseling
- chronic pain syndromes

[3]Quality management
- chart review
- critical paths
- variance analysis
- statistical analysis
- health outcomes measurement
- team building
- literature review

[4]Specialty case management
- high-risk maternity
- chronic renal failure
- asthma
- hemophilia
- geriatric
- forensic
- HIV+/AIDS
- acquired brain injury

[5]Alternative/holistic practices
- therapeutic touch
- massage therapy
- guided meditation
- Tai Chi

[6]Utilization management
- build phone relationships
- anticipate clinical problems
- manage many issues at once

the skill set to move into another area of practice, they can look for ways to move to that setting. If they are lacking a skill required for the new setting, they can find out if there are opportunities for training in that skill.

Assessing People Skills

The Thomas-Kilmann Conflict Mode Instrument is a commercially available psychometric survey instrument that is helpful to people who need feedback on their conflict resolution skills.[2] It profiles an individual's behavioral propensity in conflict situations along two basic dimensions: assertiveness, the extent to which a person attempts to satisfy his or her own concerns, and cooperativeness, the extent to which the person attempts to satisfy other people's concerns. Five modes of behavior are identified: competing (forcing), collaborating (problem solving), compromising (sharing), avoiding (withdrawal), and accommodating (smoothing). The instrument gives scores in relation to an average derived from the preferred mode of behavior of people in business management positions when they are faced with conflict.

Competing behavior is assertive and uncooperative. Those who pursue their own goals at the expense of others are generally identified as powerful people. They use their power to advance or defend their position. A competition mode is best used when quick, decisive action is vital, such as in an emergency department.

Accommodating behavior is unassertive and cooperative—the opposite of competing behavior. An accommodating person neglects his or her own concerns to satisfy the concerns of others. Accommodators may accept another's suggestions, whether they personally agree or not. This style is best used by those who realize that they themselves may be wrong and want to allow a better position to be heard, showing that they are reasonable and willing to learn from others.

Avoiding behavior is unassertive and uncooperative. Avoiders do not address the conflict. Instead, they postpone action and shun confrontation. Avoiding behavior is appropriate when the issue is trivial or when more important issues are pressing.

Collaborating behavior is assertive and cooperative—the opposite of avoiding behavior. Collaborators attempt to work with others to find solutions that fully satisfy the concerns of both persons. Often, this approach requires digging into the underlying issues to find alternatives that meet both sets of concerns. Collaborating is best used when both sets of concerns are too important to be compromised and an integrative solution may make it possible to address the concerns of all parties.

Compromising behavior is intermediate in both assertiveness and cooperativeness. An expedient, mutually acceptable solution that partially satisfies both parties is the goal of the compromiser. Compromising gives up more than competing, but less than accommodating. This form of conflict resolution is best used when goals for each side are of only moderate importance and not worth the effort or potential disruption of more assertive action.

Success in some work situations and career choices demands certain types of behaviors from people. Different conflict resolution skills are needed in different settings and at different times. People successful at resolving conflict tend to know what their basic style is and can adjust their style to fit the situation. This self-knowledge of conflict resolution skills can be an important factor in choosing a practice setting or the kind of training or skill set necessary for success.

Recognizing an Entrepreneur's Skill Set

For some people, the lure of self-employment can be very enticing. Not everyone has the temperament to own and operate a business or even to be a manager, however. Table 4–1 shows the differing styles of behavior characteristic of a technical expert who leaves certain details to others, a manager, and an entrepreneur.

Training for Skill Set

Individuals may acquire those skills that are essential for a targeted job or professional position, but not part of their repertoire, through training, either formal or informal. Recently, a psychiatric nurse in an inpatient facility sought advice because she was worried about losing her job. The facility was unable to keep its beds full and was having difficulty collecting from insurance companies for services rendered. She thought case management sounded like a nice change of pace. Because she did not have many skills that she could immediately bring to the work force, other than her position at the psychiatric hospital, her counselor urged her to volunteer for the committees at her facility that were concerned with quality im-

Table 4–1 Characteristics of Differing Business Behavioral Styles

Technician	Manager	Entrepreneur
Doer/Know-how	Pragmatic	Visionary
Ruminates on past	Present focused	Future focused
Individualist	Needs order	Needs control
Practical thinking	Tactical thinking	Strategic thinking
Likes status quo	Likes status quo	Likes change
Sees solutions	Sees problems	Sees opportunities

Source: Compiled in part from M.E. Gerber, *The Myth Revisited,* © 1995, Harper Collins Publishers, Inc.

provement and utilization management. She asked for training in the coding of diagnoses and procedures, the process of utilization management, and the reasons for the insurers' denials of benefits. She found out as much as she could about the payers (behavioral management companies) and their policies and procedures. This would give her a starting point for training herself and enhancing her skill set in an area about which she already knows a great deal.

What this nurse learned was that behavioral management companies are either owned or contracted by insurance companies to do claims management (i.e., adjudicate all requests for service and review bills and pay them) for any patient requiring behavioral health services (i.e., treatment for psychiatric disturbances or drug or alcohol abuse). She learned how referrals are made, what each payer's criteria were regarding approval for proposed services, and the billing and reporting expectations for each payer. She learned that each payer had counselors on the other end of the phone who were psychiatric nurses. She learned that her psychiatric hospital and the psychiatrists were not prepared to systematically answer questions about rationale for the proposed services, and the intensity and outcome of the services that the payer was looking for. The nurse began to catalogue the payers' responses to requests for service, and she even identified individuals with whom she had repeated contact. This enabled her to understand what language should be used when service requests and reauthorization for service requests were made for specific payers. The result was an improvement in payment for services rendered by the facility, an improvement in her value to her employer, and an improvement in her satisfaction with her work. Furthermore, her suggested changes in the format of the medical record progress notes made the records easier to understand for all the therapists in her hospital.

Notes

Insights that she gained also helped her to contribute suggestions about a halfway house service that the hospital was considering for patients who previously would have become inpatients but were now denied those more expensive services.

Networking To Enhance Skill Set

Joining local chapters of professional organizations is another way for people to enhance their skill set and meet others who have similar interests. The local chapters are often very active and inexpensive, and they all need members who can help with the organization's activities: programs, newsletters, sales of exhibit space to sponsors/vendors, membership, bylaws, and hospital functions. Skills practiced include:

- forming group consensus and running group meetings
- making up budgets
- projecting revenue
- contacting speakers and sponsors
- applying for continuing education credits
- making up brochures
- obtaining mailing lists
- arranging for conference space
- negotiating prices
- planning exhibit space
- obtaining publicity
- keeping membership lists
- maintaining financial records

Skill sets are learned without pressure under these circumstances. No one cares if a new member does not do everything right the first time; after all, it is a volunteer organization. Further, those who join these organizations are also likely to be interested in the career advancement opportunities available. They are glad to share what they know and are grateful for the assistance of interested members.

Contacts gained through networking in local professional organizations do not show an immediate payoff. The payoff comes with time, as members change jobs and as the market changes. Thus, the time to start networking is *before* being downsized.

Getting a Coach

Some skills are discrete. They demand a coach, someone who can help other people develop themselves in a step-by-step way as they practice and strive to improve. Many professionals already know this; for example, actors hire voice coaches, dance coaches, professional trainers, makeup artists, wardrobe specialists, and so forth. They plan success, and they carry out plans. Success is not a matter of luck or happenstance.

Coaching can be informal, such as advice from friends. In this case, however, the coach or advisor (i.e., friend) may not be in a position to comment expertly on a person's ability or change in style. The friend may not be available when needed most. A coach whom clients interview, check the references of, and pay within a specified agreement or contract has much more value. Such coaches are asked to set aside their personal agendas and devote their attention to the client's needs. They have a reputation to maintain, and a satisfied customer may be able to refer more business to them. If they are well-known in their field, they may also be a very good source of employment referrals.

CREDENTIALS

At a time when the whole health care delivery system is in a state of flux and practices are changing daily, credentials become more important than ever. Organizations require staff who are credentialed because their customers want to see evidence of staff expertise. Credentialing bodies (e.g., the Joint Commission on Accreditation of Healthcare Organizations, National Commission for Quality Assurance, Commission for Accreditation of Rehabilition Facilities), regulators, and payers (e.g., insurance companies, managed care organizations) need to report to *their* credentialing and regulatory bodies on their efforts to ensure high-quality service. Therefore, any practice credential that health care providers can obtain is worth the money and effort.

Advanced education credentials are also important, because regulatory bodies want to see evidence of expertise. Nurses should investigate degree programs to ensure that they choose the right one for them. For anyone who plans to stay in nursing, a nursing degree enhances flexibility. Not all nursing programs are alike. Many have excellent reputations among the students who have attended; many others are offering distance learning opportunities. Anyone who wants to attend school can probably find a program that offers the style of instruction and specialty training desired.

CONCLUSION

There are many different types of skills needed for personal and career success. Nurses get a quick snapshot of their skills and proficiencies by analyzing their work histories and the technical and people skills they have acquired. The nursing skill set matrix is an additional worksheet that aids in sorting out which skills have been acquired and in what settings they may be useful.

Important components for success in the emerging marketplace include problem identification and problem solving, information finding and information systems, and negotiating skills with people, including coaching and counseling skills. The highest paid and most valued workers are symbolic analysts, who are adept at systems thinking and have a number of skill sets, both technical skills and people skills.

Those who lack proficiency in a necessary skill area need to get training or coaching in that skill. Different people and situations require various types of skills; for example, entrepreneurs and people in business have different skill needs than clinicians. Networking itself is a skill, and joining professional organizations may enable a person to enhance his or her skill set in a safe environment. Earning educational or certification credentials can distinguish a person who is seeking advancement in certain growing fields.

NOTES

1. R. Reich, *The Work of Nations* (New York: Knopf, 1994).
2. K. Thomas and R. Kilmann, *Thomas-Kilmann Conflict Mode Instrument* (Tuxedo, NY: Xicom, 1974).

5

Case Management:
A Practice Model
for the Future

The concept of case management by nurses makes sense in the age of managed care. It makes sense from the payer point of view because it focuses on those patients most likely to require a great many resources. Proper "management" of each case can anticipate problems and adjust care processes for selected diagnoses. It makes sense from the patient point of view because many patients do better if someone can guide them through the system. Nurses are in the best position to provide this type of service because they have an understanding of how the health system works and they can address medical as well as social and practical issues with patients, families, insurance companies, lawyers, and physicians. Except for some hospital, health maintenance organization (HMO), and community nursing programs, acceptance of nursing case management is still evolving.

HISTORY OF CASE MANAGEMENT

Case management has been around for many years. Social workers and community health nurses used this approach in the early part of the century. Insurance-based case management began after World War

II with workers' compensation patients; later, group health, long-term disability, and automobile insurance carriers began to use rehabilitation case managers to coordinate the care of the catastrophically injured or ill as part of a cost containment effort. More recently, HMOs and occupational health nurses have coordinated the care of patients who require complex care or are chronically ill. Special programs for Medicare and Medicaid patients are also using the case management model for selected patients (e.g., older people who are frail, those who are blind, children with severe disabilities, patients with acquired brain injuries).

Hospitals began to use the term *case management* to describe a way to manage diagnostically selected patients within the institutions so as to decrease length of stay and reduce costs. This use of the term has caused some confusion as to its meaning. *Case management* focuses on single patients and specifies patient-specific outcomes. *Care management,* what hospitals do, is process focused; by using treatment algorithms (e.g., critical paths, clinical paths, CareMAPs), it strives to improve the efficiency and effectiveness of the care provided for diagnostically chosen patients. Further, care management is generally directed toward patients within a specific setting, whereas case management is intended to coordinate care as the patient moves from acute care to rehabilitation to home or nursing facility. Case managers also manage patients who are in the home setting so as to reduce the need for inpatient care, thus both saving money and maintaining the patient's health-related quality of life.

COST CONTAINMENT EFFORTS IN MANAGED CARE

Risk sharing arrangements involve contractual agreements regarding a provider's payment per member per month. A portion of this, typically 20 percent, goes into a "risk pool" that is held in escrow. The provider whose practice is consistent with predetermined utilization guidelines eventually receives the escrow funds. Physicians who exceed their utilization quotas because, for example, their patients required longer than expected hospitalizations, may have their HMO contract abrogated. Some HMOs can do this without specifying the cause, although several states are now passing legislation to curtail this practice. More often, providers who do not meet the utilization guidelines do not receive all their escrow funds or are asked to attend educational sessions to review the best practice expectations of the insurer.

Some managed care organizations (MCOs) use discounted fee-for-service fee schedules and aggressive utilization management to preauthorize diagnostic and surgical procedures, as well as inpatient stays. In one emerging method of risk sharing, the MCO gives an integrated delivery system a percentage of the monthly fee that it collects from the payer. If the MCO collects $500 per subscriber per month on a Medicare contract, for example, it pays a provider organization a flat fee of $350 ($500 × .70) per month to provide all the medical services that the subscriber may need. If the MCO receives more money from the payer, the monthly payment to the provider rises. If the MCO receives less, the monthly fee to the provider decreases. Thus, as competition increases in areas of heavy market penetration by MCOs, the price of coverage may decrease, thus decreasing reimbursement to providers in the future.

Case Management for Controlling Costs

Case management is one of the repertoire of cost containment and quality improvement strategies that insurance companies (including HMOs, self-funded employers, and union-funded health insurance) and integrated delivery systems that take on risk contracts use in trying to provide appropriate benefits while meeting their legal and financial contract obligations.

Managing health care is a function of knowing the probable rate of utilization and monitoring the actual rate of utilization against the expected norm. Although case managers are valuable in closely managing high-risk, high-cost cases, it does not make economic sense to attempt to manage the costs of all patient utilization.

Having identified certain common diagnoses that may require costly care, MCOs can anticipate such aspects of care as the tests, medications, and number of office visits necessary to treat the identified diagnosis effectively. They monitor treatment in relation to the expected norm and collect data on practice patterns for providers. They then analyze the data collected in comparison to other data, such as patient satisfaction, hospitalization rate, and length of stay, to arrive at a profile of the provider. This analysis determines the provider's future relations with the MCO (e.g., the payout from the risk pool).

Provider organizations (e.g., hospitals, integrated delivery systems, physician group practices, subacute care centers) should collect data about the patient, including the diagnosis, comorbidities, the intensity of service, the cost of care, and patient satisfaction. These data need to be analyzed internally not only to anticipate the feedback from the MCO, but also to identify areas of potential improvement within the organization. Such areas can involve business processes as well as clinical processes.

Contrary to the intuitive feelings of many clinicians, higher quality care *can* be achieved with lower costs. Efficient business processes eliminate many of the reasons for redoing laboratory tests and other procedures (due to lost results or incorrect reports); effective medical recordkeeping helps prevent miscommunications among clinicians and denial of payment by insurance companies. Clinicians who value efficient and standardized business functioning are comfortable proceeding with diagnosis and treatment that are focused and based on best practice algorithms. Although algorithms take away a certain amount of choice from physicians and other clinicians, their use fosters the identification of data elements (discrete information useful in measuring the effectiveness of treatment) that can lead to improvements in rendering medical care and other health care interventions.

Return on Investment

Insurance companies, self-funded employers, and other payers want to know about the efficiency and effectiveness of care. They want data that show them the value of the health care services rendered. The value of the service is usually calculated as a dollars spent divided by dollars saved ratio. For example, what is the amount of money saved by a large employer who has a special program for avoiding repetitive-motion injuries (e.g., carpal tunnel syndrome) in the workplace? The calculation would be the total savings of medical payments, sick time, and payment to replace the injured workers before the program versus the total after the program is started, divided by the total cost of the program. Often, provider organizations cannot provide cost data on specific diagnoses so that costs can be compared for patients with same or similar diagnoses. Return on investment is a calculation of costs versus benefits. Another way to use return on investment is to assist in judging the merit of proposals for alternative treatment plans. In terms of a return-on-investment strategy, what is the relative benefit of the various proposed treatment plans? Further, what does the patient believe will work best for him or her? A plan that the patient believes in or values has a better chance of success.

The general calculation of the value of case management services is:

$$\frac{\text{Cost of care without case management}}{\text{Cost of care with case management}}$$

This can be calculated with single patients or groups of patients within specific diagnostic categories.

Table 5–1 illustrates the cost of care in a case management program for asthmatic children. Before case management, the costs incurred included physician office visits, emergency department visits, medication, and hospitalizations (incidence and length of stay). After the initiation of case management, all these costs decreased; however, there was a cost for the case management itself. The return on investment became

$$\frac{\text{Cost of care without case management}}{\text{New costs} + \text{cost of case management}}$$

Return on investment may involve hard and soft savings. Hard savings are generally those gained by negotiating a decrease in the price of services or equipment, or by finding a way to obtain services for free or to shift the cost of services to another insurance carrier or the social service system. Soft savings can be more problematic. Case management may be instituted only after the treatment plan has failed more than once (e.g., for someone having chronic pain). A case manager who changes the treatment plan and is successful can point to the fact that the cost of services decreased after case management. The savings are called soft savings, however, because the

Table 5–1 Return on Investment for an Asthma Case Management (CM) Program for Children

Type of Service	Cost Pre-CM ($)	Cost Post-CM ($)	% Change
Physician office visits (@$60/per)	72,000	36,000	−50
Medications (includes oral steroids and antibiotics)	142,000	56,800	−60
Emergency department visits (@$1,500)	315,000	157,580	−50
Hospitalizations (@$5,400)	486,000	320,760	−34
Total	1,015,000	571,140	
Cost of case management (300 × $390)	0	117,000	
Total costs with case management		688,140	−32
Savings		326,860	

Return on investment for case management: $326,860/$117,000 = $2.79/$1.00

individual may not have required the same services under case management that he or she required before case management became involved. Soft savings are generally reported to insurance companies who contract with case management on a case-by-case basis.

USE OF THE CASE MANAGER'S SKILL SET TO IMPROVE OUTCOME

The case manager translates the patient's priorities, the payer's priorities, and the proposed treatment plans into strategies for the future treatment of the patient. Using the leadership skills of listening, analyzing, coaching, and counseling, the case manager looks at the patient's needs in a way that differs from that of the traditional nurse. Generally, nurses are taught and socialized to assess the patient's needs and to take care of those needs for the patient. In contrast, case managers attempt to help the patient and family assume the responsibility of their own care.

Modern case management comes from a rehabilitation focus. Case managers originally oversaw the treatment course of severely injuried patients as they worked their way through the health care system. In guiding the care from acute hospitalization, to inpatient rehabilitation, to home and outpatient rehabilitation, case managers became aware of the need to foster a sense of independence in their patients. While striving to do transferable skills assessments and other vocational counseling, these case managers learned how to help patients identify and set personal goals, break down the steps to achievement of those goals, and work toward the achievement of those goals. Because they have been forced to negotiate for the costs of equipment, hospitalization, and therapy, case managers have learned to function in the world of business. Their emphasis on the value of self-responsibility encouraged patients and their families to learn about the insurance system, the health care system, the social service system, and even some aspects of the legal system so that they could reach their goals.

SETTINGS OF CASE MANAGEMENT

Case managers who are generally recognized to practice within an institution or organization are called internal case managers. Those who manage the patient from outside the provider setting are called external case managers. Case managers can be paid by the insurance company, the patient/family, the government, or another payer. The position of case management and the identity of the payer can determine the effectiveness or leverage that the case manager has with the providers and the patient.

Internal Case Management

An internal case manager oversees the patient's care while the staff nurse follows the critical path. The case manager has no hands-on responsibilities but anticipates discharge needs, answers insurance inquiries, coordinates efficient treatment interventions, and collects data to aid with quality improvement initiatives. Thus, while the staff nurse monitors the critical path (if in place) and the patient's progress in relation to an expected length of stay, the internal case manager assumes more of a quality focus. The internal case manager collects and tracks data on such aspects of care as cost, utilization, patient and family satisfaction, and services denied. Although the collection of these data may be an anathema to many bedside nurses, it plays an important role in the institution's survival. This quality function also should include training in using the data to drive programmatic changes.

Social Service Model of Hospital Case Management

Some hospital case management programs have a social service/discharge planning function. Discharge to a more appropriate setting reduces length of stay but seems to be an avoidance of loss for a single facility rather than a gain for the system. Some hospitals have reduced or eliminated the social service staff because patients are no longer in the hospital long enough to require the traditional counseling skills of a social worker.

Social workers' knowledge of the social service system, particularly what determines the eligibility for county welfare system and the Medicare and Medicaid programs, is an important part of stretching resources within a hospital or nursing home. In many cases, however, social workers who make placements to long-term care facilities do not pass along enough information to the nursing staff that is responsible for admitting the patient. The resulting miscommunication can be costly to all involved: the patient, family, sending/receiving institutions, physician, and payer. Even so, social workers have an important supportive role as part of any case management effort.

Clinical Specialists as Case Managers

Nurses with advanced clinical skills (e.g., clinical specialists or nurse practitioners) who have the respect of the physicians and house staff can be especially effective in the role of case manager. They may assist individual physician practices or hospital departments by coordinating patient admissions, discharges, and follow-up care. In many hospitals, the nurse case manager may also act as a coach and counselor to the patient and family. Some may have assignments to call discharged patients to check on their status, especially high-risk patients, such as the frail elderly.

Internal case managers who are clinical specialists may also have a role in educating payers about special diagnoses or patient circumstances. Specialty hospitals may have their case managers meet with payer utilization management nurses to share their respective rationales regarding denials of payment for care proposed or rendered.

Intermediate and Long-Term Care Case Managers

Internal case managers in subacute, rehabilitation, and long-term care facilities not only have the responsibilities of case management, but also act as admission liaisons and marketing representatives for the facility. They need to know about the quality of their institution, the types of insurance, the preferences of the various insurance companies, and referral sources. They need to communicate well with all types of personalities—distraught families, distracted physicians, cognitively impaired patients, overworked insurance claims representatives, and so on.

Any health care organization, such as an HMO, a physician practice group, a psychiatric or behavioral health clinic, or an occupational health setting, may find an internal case manager helpful. In each of these settings, the needs of the stakeholders of the organization define the role of the case manager. In addition, the case manager should look for new ways to demonstrate the value of case management activity.

External Case Management

In general, external case management involves managing the patients as they traverse systems or sites of care. External case managers understand how the health care system operates, what the priorities of the insurance company or payer are, and how competing concerns of the various parties can be balanced. External case managers may be employed by insurance companies or independent case management firms. They may also contract with the insurer, the patient, or personal injury lawyers to manage cases involving high-cost, chronic conditions or catastrophic injuries. They are often charged with investigating as well as managing the case.

Some external case managers work for an insurance company or subcontract through an independent case management company. Others are self-employed, working for a host of different insurance companies, personal injury lawyers, unions, or employers who may be self-insured for their workers' compensation or health insurance.

External case managers need to be able to present themselves to physicians, patients, lawyers, court officers, and insurance company representatives in person. They need telephone skills to obtain vital information from medical records departments, physicians' offices, internal case managers, and others—all of whom have different procedures about releasing patient records and may have different views of case management. They need to have sources to describe and explain the appropriate treatment plans for many different kinds of complex cases involving rare diseases and multiple, catastrophic injuries.

CERTIFICATION ISSUES FOR CASE MANAGERS

The Commission for Case Manager Certification held its first certifying examination in May 1993. Although the certified case manager (CCM) credential is thought to be very clinically oriented, it also requires knowledge of insurance systems, alternative funding sources, and social service systems (e.g., Medicare, Medicaid). Before they can become CCMs, practitioners must have a license or certification to practice independently in their field, such as nursing; social service; physical, occupational, or speech therapy; or psychological services. Their job descriptions must indicate that they perform all the components of case management as defined by the Case Management Society of America: assessment, planning, coordination, implementation, monitoring, and evaluation activities for the sick and injured.[1] Further, they may practice in various settings.

Other credentials are also available to case managers; among them are the following:

- Certified Professional in Healthcare Quality (CPHQ). The National Association for Healthcare Quality certifies primarily those quality assurance/improvement professionals in hospitals, although it recognizes the important role of those who construct critical paths to make the care more efficient and effective. This is a very good credential for those involved with quality improvement.

- Certified Disability Management Specialist (CDMS), formerly Certified Insurance Rehabilitation Specialist (CIRS). Offered by the Commission for Case Manager Certification, this credential is for vocational or rehabilitation counselors. The focus is on vocational assessment, disability issues, and rehabilitation services and care. This credential is very useful in states with workers' compensation laws that emphasize vocational rehabilitation after an injury.

CONCLUSION

Case and care management positions are growing at a rapid pace, although the pay, training, and status is not increasing at the same pace. Case management is an important model for the future of nursing practice, however, as it involves assisting patients as they move through the health care system. Case managers need to have a good understanding of the clinical issues and the system characteristics related to the patients with whom they are involved. This area of practice can be very gratifying because of the independent nature of the practice and the continuity of care involved.

NOTE

1. "Commission for Case Manager Certification," *CCM Certification Guide* (Rolling Meadows, IL: Commission for Case Manager Certification, 1996).

Part II

Dynamics of Personal Empowerment

Personal empowerment is your ability to improve the quality of your life through a continuous process of personal expansion, exploration, and emotional development.

We are all endowed with the potential to create opportunity, overcome adversity, and contribute to humanity. We have one life to discover our destiny and fulfill it. What we do with that gift is a decision each of us must live with.

INTRODUCTION

Part I of this book was designed to induce a sense of constructive discontent in the reader, a sense of restlessness that will motivate reading and working with the real substance of this book, contained in the chapters that follow. Part II is designed to guide readers through the steps of change, or transition from their old selves to the new beings that the readers will invent. The methods described herein require groundwork and careful consideration over time to enhance the value of the innovative thinking that the reader can develop.

Each person has an ideal life and work situation that can become real if the necessary work is accomplished that makes it real. Time must be set aside each day to construct the lists and practice mental habits defined in these chapters that can lead to success in personal and professional endeavors. The methodology described is one that has worked for many people, but it usually requires the construction of a personal support system that will help make the goals more real and the motivation stronger.

6

Personal Transitions

The dictionary defines *transition* as the passing from one condition, place, or activity to another. It is a much more complex and time-consuming process than change. For example, painting and buying new furniture would be a change; however, moving from an apartment to a home in another town, with new schools, a new neighborhood, and a new lifestyle is a transition. Thus, a transition requires a mental and emotional adjustment over a period of time. It may also mean an adjustment of personal identity. If personally chosen, a transition could be a tremendous boost to self-esteem; if mandated by a shift in environment (as with nurses and managed care), it could make an individual question his or her self-worth.

PROACTIVE VS. REACTIVE TRANSITION

In a proactive transition, the individuals in transition recognized or created an opportunity for positive change and positioned themselves to make the move. The transition was born from a constructive discontent with the status quo. They may have been planning it for months or even years, and now it is time to

121

make the move. The energy and excitement compensate for the doubt and the fear of any unknowns. Therein lies a sense of personal control over destiny.

In contrast, individuals in a reactive transition feel more like victims than victors. This type of transition can be devastating or even immobilizing, depending on the level of surprise or expectation of the transition. If it was completely unforeseen, such as a layoff from a long-term, comfortable job situation, a reactive transition can produce monumental emotional turmoil. This is very similar to a sudden separation in a marriage, where one partner has no clue that the other is leaving until the departure. Many psychologists working with people who have found themselves unemployed because of corporate downsizing say it is not unusual for these clients to identify themselves by the job title they lost six months ago.

STAGES OF TRANSITION

The length of the person's awareness of the oncoming transition and the depth of the person's ability to adjust to drastic changes determine at what level that person will move through the three stages of transition.

The Ending

The initial stage of transition is called the "ending." Because the transition involves the loss of the present situation and identity, the person goes through a process that is very similar to the natural grieving process associated with the death of a loved one. The typical stages of grieving are

1. initial shock and immobilization
2. denial

3. anger
4. bargaining
5. grief
6. eventual acceptance

People in transition may at first feel immobilized or overwhelmed, unable to understand what is happening or determine what steps should be taken next. There may be a feeling of panic or a loss of energy. People have been known to move into denial to minimize the impact of a loss, not accepting that the change is really happening. They may create false hope for themselves. Sometimes, they use a great deal of energy to maintain the illusion of the past reality. Often, depression sets in, followed by frustration coupled with a devasting sense of loss. Eventually, they realize that things have changed and will never be the same. They are not sure yet how to cope. The emotional roller coaster has not stopped, and their energy is nearly drained.

The Neutral Zone

The second stage of transition is the state that lies between the old and the new reality—the "neutral zone." It can be a time of confusion with major shifts between hopefulness and despair. It is an incubation period that holds an abundance of creative potential and new ideas. During this time, people in transition slowly let go of outdated beliefs and expectations. They begin to accept the reality that the old ways no longer exist. As they move through this process, their energy begins to increase. Hope finds its way back into their life as they begin testing new ideas. Moments of enthusiasm occur. Some time is spent in contemplation as they try to understand what the previous phases have meant. The past and the present start to merge as these individuals look into all the possibilities for their future. Overall, their energy flow comes back as they consider new beginnings.

The New Beginnings

Identified as "new beginnings," the third stage of transition is the acceptance of past events and the incorporation of a new sense of reality. It involves new visions that come to light after the old visions have been put to rest. These ideas are built on the new orientations of personal identity and opportunity that emerge in the neutral zone. A new sense of personal identity converts itself into emotion and behavior. Optimism replaces depression because of the acceptance of the new reality. With renewed hope for the future comes a rejuvenation of energy resources. As self-confidence returns, it increases the person's ability to generate new ideas for his or her life.

Transition Timeline

Both the circumstances that bring on the transition and timeline itself are different for different people. Further, stages may overlap as people move from one stage to the next. As Figure 6–1 illustrates, people may

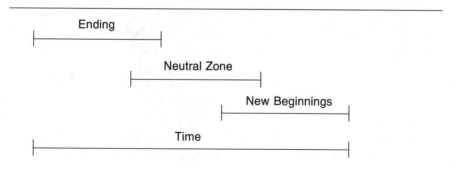

Figure 6–1 Timeline graph for transition

vacillate as they move through the process. A person who would like to move forward more quickly or has remained in one place too long may find personal counseling or a support group helpful.

THE HAMMER THAT SHATTERS THE GLASS FORGES THE STEEL

The circumstances in which people find themselves do not *define* who they are—circumstances *reveal* who they are. Events may certainly have an influence, but it is their response to these events that determines the outcome. It may be a cliché, but problems are indeed opportunities in disguise (Exhibit 6–1). Behind each problem is a gift; the person who solves the problem

---

Exhibit 6–1 What Is Life?

> **What Is Life?**
>
> *Life Is a Challenge . . . Meet It*
> *Life Is a Gift . . . Accept It*
> *Life Is an Adventure . . . Explore It*
> *Life Is a Sorrow . . . Overcome It*
> *Life Is a Tragedy . . . Face It*
> *Life Is a Game . . . Play It*
> *Life Is a Mystery . . . Unfold It*
> *Life Is a Song . . . Sing It*
> *Life Is an Opportunity . . . Take It*
> *Life Is a Journey . . . Complete It*
> *Life Is a Promise . . . Fulfill It*
> *Life Is a Rainbow . . . Find It*
> *Life Is a Struggle . . . Fight It*
> *Life Is a Goal . . . Achieve It*
> *Life Is a Puzzle . . . Solve It*
> *Life Is a Celebration . . . Enjoy It*
> *Life Is a Lesson . . . Learn It*
> *Life Is a Love . . . Embrace It*

Source: Copyright © Irv Furman.

receives the gift. The gift has many variations: a solution, a positive outcome, wisdom, experience, knowledge, or a stronger character. One woman has a great response when someone asks how she is doing when she is having a bad day: "I'm having a character-building day." The stress of such days makes it possible to stretch the imagination along with so many other talents and abilities that will ultimately build confidence and self-esteem.

DEPTH OF THE HUMAN SPIRIT

There are people who have bounced back from great adversity in their lives. The initial shock, denial, depression, and fear forced these people to deal with the feelings of emotional turmoil that they must endure before they stabilize their feelings. Somehow, for example, many people who become disabled as a result of an unfortunate accident find the strength, courage, and determination to resume functioning at a level that allows them to lead a normal life. A select few go even further to accomplish great things in spite of their handicap. The Para-Olympics is a perfect example of such courage through adversity.

Self-Dignity

The resources for such power lie deep in the heart of everyone. There seems to be an energy source of hidden strength and determination that comes along with something that can be called the dignity of life. It complements a positive self-image. When people set those standards for themselves and refuse to compromise their values or priorities, the world starts to pay attention to their needs and expectations.

People who are clear about their needs and clearly believe in their abilities to meet those needs give permission for others to believe in them. At times, they will be tested, however. For example, women in self-defense workshops learn that they should never act as if they are lost, frightened, or insecure when in a strange and unknown environment. Anyone looking for a victim goes for the weakest one first.

Both verbal and nonverbal communications reveal much about a person's level of self-confidence. Following are just a few indicators of self-confidence:

- responsibility taken for personal actions
- voice inflection, eye contact, body language
- behavior when right
- behavior when wrong
- attitude toward criticism
- ability to deal with setbacks
- treatment of people in authority
- treatment of people without authority
- composure when questioned about abilities
- projection of inner peace or security

Value of Self-Esteem

More opportunities come to those who believe that they can handle those opportunities. These people seem to be comfortable with who they are. They know where they want to go and why they want to go there, they have a plan to get there, and they believe they are going to make it. This creates the desire either to help them or to get out of their way. These individuals have a charisma, an air of confidence, an attraction.

Custom-Designing Your Life

The remaining chapters of this book are about reinventing one's career by custom-designing one's life. The key is to custom-design one's identity and to visualize the desired direction of one's life. Transition can force a person out of the nest. The stage of transition being experienced (ending, neutral, or new beginnings) may determine the level of enthusiasm for the task. The principles, tools, and processes in the following chapters are designed to provide the opportunity to make choices about the most important things in life and to keep on making the right choices until one feels satisfied with the quality of life that has been created. At that point, belief in oneself and confidence in the process may bring even higher levels of achievement.

The Good News

Now is the moment to shine! By the time people reach adulthood, they get about 50 years to see what they can accomplish. That's 50 years to see what is possible with this thing called life. There are no dress rehearsals. Consider all the people who were at the top of their game 10, 20, and 30 years ago. Where are they now? What could they accomplish now if they wanted to? They took advantage of this opportunity called life when they had the chance. Certainly, it got a little stressful at times, but do they have regrets now? The lesson to be learned is seize the moment of opportunity to experience life at its fullest.

The Bad News

Personal growth may equal pain—but it's a good pain. Let's compare the pain of a physical injury with the pain of physical exercise. One is an unhealthy kind of pain, and the other is a healthy kind of pain. The pain endured by creating opportunity in life and making it happen is not the pain of poverty or sickness. It is the pain that happens when those mental and emotional muscles are stretched to the utmost. One of the best antidotes to the pain of personal growth is for people to develop a sense of humor about themselves and their mistakes. Most people take their life goals too lightly and take themselves too seriously. This creates mediocrity because, for fear of failing and looking foolish, people talk themselves out of trying to achieve their personal goals. This can be a fatal error and a dream killer. People must learn to have a good laugh at themselves. A sense of humor is often a person's most underused natural resource.

7

The Process of Personal Empowerment

Personal empowerment is the ability to improve the quality of life through a continuous process of personal expansion, exploration, and emotional development. Thus, empowerment is a journey, a process, an adventure, a purpose and a calling, a vision, a mission, and a responsibility. It is being willing to step out of the comfort zone and into the pain zone to reach the end zone. It is life at full blast and having a blast. It goes beyond making a living. It is creating a lifestyle. It is applying imagination and choosing courage as an option when needed. It means not always following a well-worn path but, at times, choosing a new path and leaving a trail.

FORCES OF EMPOWERMENT

The world is full of powerful natural forces, and Mother Nature is not unlike any other loving mother. Those who understand and follow her guidelines in life will find wellness, happiness, and even prosperity. Those who misuse her principles, however, can make things very difficult for themselves.

Gravity, for example, is a basic force of nature. It keeps people in place; it is stable and predictable.

Understanding the principles of gravity makes it possible to do wonderful things, like fly, but its misuse could be life-threatening. Human habits are a great deal like gravity. They keep people heading on a specific or certain course. They are stable and predictable. Positive habits can lead anywhere desired. Negative habits can bring all progress to a halt and the result could be self-destructive.

The forces of empowerment are the external natural laws and principles that nature offers as systems, guidelines, tools, and natural phenomena to determine the "gravity" of human life. Being aware of their availability is the first major step. Choosing to act upon them and direct them is a choice each person has to make.

Change itself is a force of empowerment. People need to give up the comfort of thinking that they cannot change. The question is not whether to change, but *how* to change. Most individuals do not realize that they are in a constant state of change and it is their responsibility to drive that change. Driving that change in the direction of their dreams will provide them with the key to a happy, productive life. They need to look back to life five years ago—what priorities, goals, values, and habits did they have? Ten years ago—what did they want from relationships, family, or career? People need to evaluate how their fitness and health has changed in ten years. Are their habits and behavior patterns healthier today than they were ten years ago? Is the quality of existence better now than it has ever been in life? And in how many of these changes have the individuals been proactive and in how many were they reactive?

Personal empowerment could have the same slogan as Volkswagen. "In life there are passengers and there are drivers. Drivers Wanted!" Instead, too many people have found themselves on Greyhound, "Leave the driving to us."

The greatest personal power is the power of choice. Choosing to climb into the driver's seat of life brings many responsibilities, which can be considered "response abilities." The ability of individuals to respond appropriately and in accordance with their dreams, values, priorities, and goals requires them to take the time to make conscious decisions about what things should be driving their lives. By taking the time, applying the imagination, and focusing the energy, people have the ability to become the author of their own life novel rather than just a character in someone else's script. Life is too short and too precious to settle for anything else.

THE DOUBLE-EDGED SWORD OF EMPOWERMENT

Personal empowerment is a double-edged sword. One side of that sword is the concept of the individual as the captain of his or her own ship (life), choosing to meet every challenge as an opportunity for personal growth and positive change. The other side of the sword is that the individual no longer has the option to blame everyone else for less than ideal situations. Blame has become such a big part of modern culture. The United States has become a country of blamers. Many are lawsuit crazy, pointing a finger at anyone who and anything that can help them avoid taking any personal *response ability* for the quality of their life.

According to Sykes, our culture treats lack of personal responsibility like a disease.[1] He described a phenomenon called the "medicalization of sin." Instead of taking the blame for their own wrongdoings and stupid mistakes, people turn themselves into victims. Nothing they do wrong is truly their fault because their parents made them this way or they have some sort of deficiency. They no longer make mistakes—they do wrong things because someone made them. They keep looking for other people or institutions to take responsibility for the consequences of their actions.

The U.S. Constitution does not guarantee happiness. It only offers citizens the *opportunity* to pursue happiness. It is up to them to chase it down and capture it. Happiness is their own personal state of well-being. In its pursuit, people must move forward with a vision to reach, obtain, or accomplish. So, happiness is the motivator, empowerment the process, and progress the result. The only possible limiting factor is a lack of hope or self-confidence.

FIGHT OR FLIGHT RESPONSE

One of the most basic and important natural instincts is the fight or flight response. It could propel an individual away from danger, but it could also give that individual the courage and added strength needed to take on adversaries. There is an inclination in people, just as in all animals, either to run from a crisis or to meet it head on. These feelings are still inherent in the genetic coding and the fiber of human beings. For many things, they still rely on instincts to run or stand their ground.

A perfect example of the human ability to rely on deep inner resources is Scarlett O'Hara.[2] Ms. O'Hara was the perfect debutante. Her world consisted of parties and other social occasions. She was obnoxious and stubborn. Her life goal was simple: marry rich and enjoy the good life. Then the Union Army intervened. General Sherman began his march to the sea. Scarlett saw the horrors of war as Atlanta burned before her eyes. Everything she had ever known was destroyed. All her dreams were shattered in an instant. Her sheltered life and whimsical goals had not prepared her for the cruel reality.

Finally, returning to Tara after the war, seeing all the carnage throughout Georgia, and accepting the end of her old life, Scarlett made a decision. Instead of losing all hope and running away from responsibility, she decided to take a stand. Crying out, "I'll never go hungry again!" she vowed to overcome the tragedy of war and live life with dignity and pride. She basically refused to give into the "flight" aspect of her inner self and decided to "fight" against extreme odds. A part of Scarlett lives inside everyone; many in the field of personal development refer to it as the "sleeping giant."

Life Is Ticking Away

Once a vision is created for one's life, it is time to get a sense of urgency. Here is a product that puts things in perspective: the "Life Clock." The individual programs in his or her birth date, sex, the current date, and any personal risk factors. The clock then computes the days lived and displays it on one side of the clock, and estimates how many days probably remain and displays that on the other side of the clock. Wow! This is one clock with a real wake-up call!

DEVELOPMENT OF A PERSONAL EMPOWERMENT SYSTEM

The best way to experience life with enthusiasm, optimism, and adventure is to follow nature's design for personal growth. It is a common sense approach that converts something overwhelming and complex into something simple and manageable. There is no need to do every step exactly right in the right order. That approach is guaranteed to produce frustration and *analysis paralysis*. Empowering oneself is like an author writing an exciting adventure novel. Whatever part of the book is inspiring at that moment, the author writes it. There is plenty of time to go back and fine-tune the subplots and pull it all together into a cohesive story.

The power behind the empowerment process lies in dividing life into sections and conquering them separately. Those seeking to empower themselves have an arsenal of tools available to focus, create, decide, plan, identify, and modify. They have the opportunity to customize a life by design and to avoid living a life by default. Most of what is offered in personal development is a menu of wonderful virtues to strive for with encouragement to use untapped potential and go after dreams. This system goes far beyond that. It is a step-by-step process to enable people to custom-design each area of their lives.

Use of the Life Wheel

Life can be pictured as the spokes of a wheel (Figure 7–1). Each spoke represents a significant area of life, which can be referred to as a focus area. For example, most people would identify health as an important area worth its own individual focus. Other examples are family, finances, career, recreation, spirituality, education, culture, and home. People may divide their life into as many different focus areas as necessary to fit in all the important elements of their life.

The next step is to get a three-ring binder, a set of subject dividers, and loose-leaf paper. Each divider is labeled as a spoke (i.e., focus area), and a generous amount of paper is placed behind it. (This notebook from here on out will be referred to as the Personal

Action Planner.) This arrangement makes it possible to divide each focus area of life into small enough components to identify needs clearly and to identify and modify any weaknesses. Table 7–1 lists examples of focus area subdivisions. By means of this technique, people can

- clearly isolate and focus on their needs
- create a balanced approach to life
- isolate areas of strength and weakness
- identify all components needed to support well-being

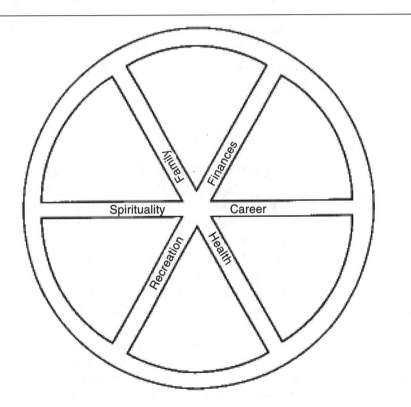

Figure 7–1 Personal life wheel. *Source:* Copyright © Achievement Dynamics Institute, Inc.

Table 7-1 Possible Focus Area Subdivisions

Family	Health	Finances
Wife Reneé	Cardiovascular exercise	Income
Daughter Maria	Weight training	Debt
Parents, in-laws	Stretching	Savings
Siblings	Balanced diet	Investments
Dog Fred	Vitamins	Expenses
Dog Barnie	Regular check-ups	Assets

- more easily create measurable objectives in the pursuit of goals
- develop life blueprints and benchmark progress

The Personal Action Planner is the nucleus of the empowerment program. This is where individuals create their life by design and write their own life novel.

Imagination and Vision

Imagination—The act or power of forming mental images of what is not actually present; creating new images by combining and learning from previous experiences.

Imagination creates visualized goals. Our imagination creates and our vision sees the creation. It has been said that no person can be any greater than his or her personal vision. Imagination is one of the human being's greatest assets. It helps people create opportunity and motivates them to find ways to make opportunity happen.

When it comes to being personally empowered, imagination is the cornerstone of success. To think creatively is to think intelligently. The men and women who are considered geniuses are not chosen by their IQ but by their creativity. Imagination multiplies all the possibilities for life. Too many people think life involves a multiple choice when, actually, activating the imagination creates *infinite choice.*

The imagination is like a muscle. It atrophies with lack of use. When asked for a wish-and-want list, no child lacks options. Unfortunately, as people grow older, they often become calloused, judgmental, and unable to see what life has to offer. Therein lies the deterioration of one of the greatest natural assets. The level in which people are empowered depends on their ability once again to expand their thinking to encompass all possibilities.

People need a breath of fresh air in the form of new ideas, new possibilities, and new approaches. It is essential to create a vision for life, to create a vision for health, relationships, and career (Exhibit 7–1).

There are several ways to stretch the imagination. A good place to start is to make a dream list, a list of all the possibilities in the heart, mind, and soul (Exhibit 7–2). There is no need to worry about whether the

---

Exhibit 7–1 A Matter of Focus

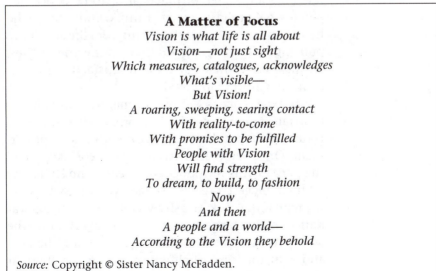

A Matter of Focus
Vision is what life is all about
Vision—not just sight
Which measures, catalogues, acknowledges
What's visible—
But Vision!
A roaring, sweeping, searing contact
With reality-to-come
With promises to be fulfilled
People with Vision
Will find strength
To dream, to build, to fashion
Now
And then
A people and a world—
According to the Vision they behold

Source: Copyright © Sister Nancy McFadden.

Exhibit 7–2 List of Dreams and Desires

Build addition on house
Get a boat
Ski the Alps
Have a "hard body"
$25,000 in savings
Take a cruise to Alaska
Average 85 golf score
Develop a retirement plan
Work in local charities
Learn to juggle
Learn CPR and first aid
Buy an in-ground pool
Build a deck in the backyard
Learn to fly
Tour Europe
Get a Harley
Become a speed-reader
Publish a book
Get a hot tub
Play the guitar
RV around the country
Meet the President

ideas are affordable or practical or to be concerned about what others may say or think. Only those who have some idea of what they want from life are able to pull together the goals that will bring the greatest enthusiasm in their pursuit and satisfaction in their achievement (Exhibit 7–3).

The experience of Kathy, a former student of mine, illustrates the success of this approach. Back in 1987, I was teaching a short course on personal empowerment. Once everyone arrived, as an icebreaker, I had the participants introduce themselves and share one of their biggest dreams. When we got to a petite woman in the back, she shyly said that her name was Kathy and her biggest dream was to travel around the world. At the end of the class, Kathy approached me and explained, in a half-whisper, that she thought she was in the wrong class and would be dropping

Exhibit 7–3 Creating Opportunities

Here are some questions to help stretch your imagination and present opportunities which could improve the quality of your life.

Which ones do you want to add to your list of possibilities?

What habits would you like to develop?
What habits would you like to break?
What personality trait would you like to develop?
What kind of home would you like to own?
What improvement would you like to make in your present home?
What vacations would you like to take?
What new position would you like to attain?
What professional or occupational skill would you like to strengthen?
What hobbies would you like to begin?
What would eliminate pressures, stresses, or worries from your life?
What specific improvements in your physical condition would you like to make?
How would you want to give back to your community?
What debts would you like to pay off?
What image would you like to communicate to others?
What are some activities you would like to do with your family?
What spiritual goals would you like to obtain?
How much money would you like to earn?
How much money would you like to save?
What physical activity would you like to start?
What things do you want to remove from your life?
What are the most important goals in: family, home, financial, career, spiritual, health, education, emotional, social, and cultural?

What is the single most important goal you would like to see accomplished in your life in the next two years?

Something so important, you can't leave it to chance.

Source: Copyright © Achievement Dynamics Institute, Inc.

out. She had mistakenly thought the class was going to be on assertiveness training, and I had never even mentioned the word during the entire class. I asked her if she had ever taken assertiveness training before. She replied, "Several times." "Did you become any more assertive?" She said, "No." I asked her if she would be willing to take a class on "assertive living." She looked confused, but she agreed to stay.

Three months after the last class, I called Kathy to see how she was doing. She enthusiastically said she was going to Australia for the entire month of July. She explained that she had noticed an advertisement in a travel magazine that said, "WANTED: Tour Guides for Australia." She recalled a principle from her empowerment class: "Those who believe they can do something and those who believe they can't, usually are both right, 100 percent of the time." Because of this, she decided to send her résumé and was subsequently hired to direct a 30-day bus tour around Australia. I said, "Kathy, I never realized you knew so much about Australia." She replied, "I don't know a darned thing about Australia, but I have two months to prepare! I am heading to the library right now to begin my research." I wished her luck.

In January of 1991, after giving a talk in the community, I was chatting with some of the folks who were there when someone tapped me on the shoulder. I turned to see Kathy. I said, "The last time we spoke, you were heading to Australia. How did you make out?" She said, "It went so well that I became a professional tour guide and, so far, in the last four years, I've been to 42 different countries."

Positive Expectancy and Optimism

The force of positive expectancy is one of the most powerful internal motivational forces. It is the belief that everything will turn out for the best. It is not enough simply to adopt a positive attitude about a particular situation and remain a pessimist about life in general. Seligman, who has done extensive research on the value of personal optimism, found that an optimistic attitude was a greater influence in success than aggressive behavior.[3]

No problem can withstand the assault of sustained thinking. People should work from the mind-set of victory, not just hope for victory. They need to see themselves as victorious over all circumstances, not a victim of circumstance. Problems are opportunities for growth. Solving the problem gives the gifts of wisdom, character, and confidence.

People who look for any kind of progress often feel encouraged; people who look for perfection often feel discouraged. Progress comes in so many different ways. The least appreciated way is through mistakes. Children learn at a very young age in school to avoid failure in any way, shape, or form. Inadvertently, many people assume that the safest way to avoid failure is to attempt nothing new. When they finally act, they magnify any little setback. Soon, the comfort zone becomes smaller and smaller. People who succeed, fail more than people who fail, however. They are able to separate themselves from their actions. If something goes wrong, they realize that their *actions* failed or fell short. They immediately start to determine how they can succeed next time. If an individual is struggling with a poor self-image, that individual takes each failure as a personal reflection of self-worth. So, the key to the learning process is to take the action believed best, evaluate the results, and make any necessary adjustments. Failure is nothing more than an opportunity to begin more intelligently.

Courage as an Option

There is a modern day parable told about two men on a tandem bike. They are biking along when they come to a steep hill in the road. It was the steepest hill either of them had ever encountered and try as they might, they could find no way around this giant obstacle. Both men were afraid that they would roll backward halfway through their climb, so with all the energy that they could muster, they raced toward the hill. Halfway up their climb, their ride became treacherous; they continued to struggle for every inch. Finally, with a final strong push, they made their way to the top of the hill. As they stopped to catch their breath, the optimist on the front of the bike proudly boasted, "It's a good thing I held the bike steady and pressed forward, or we would have fallen." The pessimist on the rear huffed back, "And it's a good thing that I held down the brakes, or we might have rolled backward!" Each person should ask himself or herself:

- Am I holding down the brakes in any area of my life?
- Am I living my life on the offense or the defense?
- Am I looking to score in the game of life, or am I just playing not to lose?
- Do I try to live by my dreams, or am I living by my fears?

Some people base decisions on fear, whereas others base decisions on opportunities.

All people have moments of doubt and fear. Those moments might cause them to lose the benefits that they would have won—had they taken the action. Because the moment of absolute certainty may never arrive, people need to be willing to deal with doubt and fear. Courage is not the absence of fear, but the conquest of it! Thus, people should live by the following guidelines:

- Don't fear criticism. If it is untrue, disregard it. If it is unfair, don't let it irritate you. If it is ignorant, smile. If it is justified, learn from it.

- Don't fear rejection. Universal acceptance does not exist.
- Don't be afraid to offer your talents, services, abilities, or friendship to others. Give people the opportunity to say yes.
- Don't fear failure. It is the ingredient essential for success. Success comes from failure. Every setback is the opportunity to move forward more intelligently and with renewed enthusiasm. Handling failure is the gateway to success.
- Don't fear change. The only consistency in life is change. Be open to it. All progress and growth comes from change.

Most fears are caused by uncertainty. To reduce fear of the unknown:

1. Write out the goals or objectives.
2. Write out the plan.
3. Write out all the benefits of success—the best scenario!
4. Write out the worst scenario in case of failure.
5. Develop a plan of action describing recovery *if* the worst-case scenario happened.
6. Determine possible improvements.

Once there was a sales team. Each individual on that team used the tools and principles of empowerment to gain success in their work. One young man named Jacob suddenly went into a deep slump. When he discussed it with his sales manager, he shared a pattern of withdrawing from his regular routine of action when he had setbacks. Jacob had recently lost two major accounts and his usual depression set in—this pattern had followed him throughout his life. The sales manager responded with a football analogy. That Sunday, the Philadelphia Eagles had played the heavily favored Washington Redskins. It was a real battle and the Eagles were losing for most of the game; then, with less than a minute to go, the Eagles ran the ball 97 yards for a touchdown and won the game. Jacob was asked if he enjoyed the game. His face lit up and the enthusiasm in his voice expressed real excitement. Then, he was asked how much he would have enjoyed the game if it were announced that the Redskins would not be showing up. In an effort not to disappoint the fans, the Eagles were still going to play, but without an opponent. Jacob looked puzzled and said, "That wouldn't be very interesting or exciting. In fact, that would be downright boring." The next question was, "Then why do you want to live your entire life with no opponents on the field? The thrill of the game is the energy, strength, endurance, and strategy that go into getting over those 11 obstacles on the field." Jacob realized that his obstacles made for a better game of life, and thus he conquered his fear of failure and became one of the most productive salespeople on the team.

Most fear comes from the unknown. People tend to assume that the unknown must automatically indicate danger or destruction. In a story about a black door, for example, a person's need to choose the known over the unknown is clear. Many years ago, the Persian Army was in the midst of a turbulent war. The jails were full of prisoners captured from the opposing army. There was no time to build additional jails, so they decided to reduce the prison population. Every morning at the crack of dawn, they randomly selected a prisoner and marched him into the courtyard for all to see. An executioner from the Persian Army then gave the prisoner two choices. The first choice was to die by the firing squad (on the left side of the courtyard there were seven Persian soldiers with high-powered rifles and a blindfold). The second choice was to pass through a mysterious, ominous black door on the right side of the courtyard. If the prisoner chose the door, he was to have been locked behind it with no way out. What was behind the black door was his fate, there was no turning back. Day after day, prisoner after prisoner chose the firing squad. One day, an aide approached the executioner and asked what lay behind the black door. "Freedom," replied the executioner. "It's amazing how so few of the prisoners choose it."

The mind takes over and plays out all the horrible things that could go wrong. Those who manage to overcome that fear and act often find out that whatever was holding them back was not really as bad as their subconscious image. Many people refer to this as False Evidence Appearing Real (FEAR). Because of FEAR, people spend too much time worrying about the problem and not enough time thinking about the solution. As Will Rogers is said to have said, "I've had a lot of problems in my life—and most of them never took place."

People need courage to choose and pursue goals that have personal meaning and worth to them. Those who take risks have doubt and fear, but they never let that doubt and fear stand in the way of the action needed to accomplish their goals. To choose courage as an option, to know that courage is not the absence of fear, but rather the conquest of it, is an essential tool in the search for empowerment in life. Courageous people are not those who are not without fear; if they were without fear, they would not need courage. The key to courage is learning to work side-by-side with fear, doubt, or uncertainty. Courage is not the easy choice, but it is a positive choice. People can draw courage from others, but no one can have courage for another. It is a choice each person must make every day.

Faith and Belief

Courage is only one step away from faith and belief in one's self, and faith and belief in a higher power. During the Dark Ages, belief in a higher power comforted people during their trials. The Renaissance belief that people could better themselves brought Medieval Europe into a new age of culture and prosperity. Having those same beliefs is essential to bouncing back from defeat and climbing up to the next level of success.

Belief in one's self energizes meaningful goals. A lack of personal belief manifests itself in a series of low-risk goals or no goals at all. People who do not think that they have what it takes may not take on the challenges needed to fight through to the next level of fulfillment. Further, belief directly affects behavior. A lack of belief in him- or herself can cause a person to accept less-than-healthy circumstances and not take the appropriate action to change them.

The most powerful belief is the belief in a higher power. People who are able to accomplish great things in life often have a sense of mission or purpose about what they do. They are able to carry greater burdens with less stress because they feel protected. They believe that if something goes wrong, help will come and their situation will work out for the best. Their belief has no limitations, because it comes from their sense of connection to their creator. For instance, in the Christian Bible, *Romans* 8:28 says, "And we all know that in all things God works for the good of those who love him who have been called according to his purpose."[4]

When people combine belief in self with belief in a higher power, it creates a powerful fusion of action with contemplation. They have the courage of their convictions to take as many steps as are necessary to achieve their purpose. So many things are possible for those who believe.

THE POWER OF ENCOURAGEMENT

Many people have launched businesses and careers, initiated relationships, or started new journeys because someone else believed in them and gave them the mental push they needed to overcome their initial fears. Like the law of physics that says a body at rest wants to stay at rest, it is necessary to overcome a tendency toward inertia to accomplish goals. On the other hand, a body in motion tends to stay in motion.

It is always important to look for ways to feel a sense of momentum. Achievement builds self-esteem, and self-esteem builds achievement. Many people keep a list of their accomplishments and achievements. At times, everyone wonders if he or she is making progress in life. A life achievement list provides proof in black and white of progress toward self-actualization.

CONCLUSION

To sum up this chapter, here are some empowerment choices that can directly affect the quality of one's life:

- I choose to be empowered.
- I choose to be proactive in who I am. The pain of becoming a complete person is essential to the joy of living.
- I choose to look at progress, not perfection.
- I choose to take responsibility, so I will respond to the best of my ability.
- I choose to realize any setback or failure is an opportunity to begin again, more intelligently.

- I choose to be optimistic and have positive expectancy.
- I choose courage as an option.
- I choose to look at my problems as opportunities for developing progress, growth, and change in who I am as a person.
- I choose to be a hero in my life novel, not a character in someone else's script.
- I choose to believe in my ability to overcome adversity and improve the quality of my life.
- I choose to live life by my own design.
- I choose the characteristics of my personality that support my vision and purposes in life.

NOTES

1. C.J. Sykes, *A Nation of Victims: The Decay of the American Character* (New York: St. Martin's Press, 1992).
2. M. Mitchell, *Gone with the Wind* (New York: Macmillan, 1936).
3. M.E. Seligman, *Learned Optimism* (New York: Alfred A. Knopf, 1990).
4. *Life Application Bible, New International Version* (Wheaton, IL: Tyndale House, 1991).

8

The Search for Answers

In the quest for the answer to life's questions, people travel many paths. Often, they have learned to believe many things that have either outlived their truthfulness, were not completely true, or were total myths from the beginning.

EDUCATION, TRAINING, AND EXPERIENCE

Education and training is a large part of the answer, but far from the only solution. Many people already possess an abundance of education, training, and experience. Chances are, they will be lucky if they use 2 percent of everything they know for the rest of their life. All that wonderful information does not guarantee a higher quality of life, however. The most empowered individuals are not necessarily the ones who have the most education, training, and experience.

In this, the information age, people have become information junkies. They want to believe the old adage, Knowledge is power. Many still believe that one more class, three more credits, or one more tape set or video just may be the answer. Gathering more information has become the path of least resistance.

151

The Internet is rapidly replacing television as the favorite means to avoid dealing constructively with the issues that people face in their lives. Education and information can be very valuable, but self-fulfillment takes kinetic power. Until it moves into action, it has very little value. Personal empowerment is about getting life into action, about setting the standards of results to a level that complements personal values, and about injecting a major dose of imagination and creativity into life. Only then is it possible to custom-design a life that will return maximum satisfaction, self-fulfillment, and inner peace.

EXTERNAL MOTIVATORS

Outside Stimulation

To *motivate* means to provide with, or affect as, a motive or motives; to incite or impel. Supposedly, if a person has the right motives and knows how to take the appropriate action, that person will be motivated. Outside sources like motivational speakers, audiotapes, videotapes, and books are all jam-packed with outstanding and life-changing powerful ideas. People may instantly feel that they can do it all, with renewed enthusiasm about their lives. But in a few days, they go right back to the same attitudes, behavior patterns, and results. Our society is caught up in what might be called the "Jack Lalane" era of personal development. In the 1960s, Jack Lalane was a popular television personality whose show was on every morning during the week. On his exercise show, Jack was the ideal model of health and fitness, saying and doing all the right things. Many people were regular viewers who listened to every word. However, when his show was over, everyone went back to their lives giving credence, but not permanence, to Jack's great suggestions. The "fix" is often only temporary, and the ideas can even become boring if heard over and over.

Fear Motivation

If there is a big enough threat to the quality of their life, people will take immediate action to avoid loss. Unfortunately, nature has an easy come, easy go, balance sheet. Fear motivation may work for a while, but humans are very adaptable creatures. They can adjust to the worst of circumstances. At best, fear motivation is temporary.

Incentive Motivation

The carrot on the end of a stick, in front of a donkey pulling a cart, works if the carrot is big enough, the stick is short enough, the cart is light enough, and the donkey is hungry enough. Change any of these variables, however, and incentive motivation stops. When it does work, the donkey must eventually get the carrot. Then, a bigger carrot, a shorter stick, or a lighter cart is necessary before the process will work again. Needless to say, as a motivational technique, incentive motivation is both tricky and temporary.

BREAKDOWN OF MOTIVATION AND TRAINING

Personal empowerment is the ability to improve the "quality of life." Many times when I am working with a new group, I ask a series of questions to help differentiate between motivation, training, and empowerment. "How many would appreciate being able to improve the quality of their life?" They all raise their hands. "How many believe that if you exercise, you will improve the quality of your health and, ultimately, the quality of your life?" Again, they all raise their hands. "So it is obvious we all have the motives to exercise. Now, if I offered you $100, how many of you could design yourself a safe and effective exercise program, without having to learn one more thing about exercise?" Almost all raise their hands. So they all have the information on how to exercise. "How many are satisfied with their current level of exercise right now?" Usually, only about 10 to 20 percent of the group raise their hands. Thus, they admitted that they have the motives and the information, but they still were not exercising. Another hour of information would be unlikely to make a difference.

How about other activities that improve the quality of life? What about time management techniques? Many people believe in and know more about personal time management than their behavior currently indicates. These same folks are the first to take another time management workshop. Communication skills? Personal goal setting? Raising positive children? Having a quality marriage? Often people attend training to hear about things they already know how to do, but just haven't managed to implement. Taking the appropiate action creates results. The key is becoming the person who takes action, transforming attitudes and habits to complement the actions necessary to attain dreams and desires. Personal change is already happening. It should be proactive, not reactive. So, the bottom line is: motivation is inspiration, training is information, and empowerment is transformation.

PROS AND CONS OF PERSONAL GOAL SETTING

The single most important ingredient in achieving a desired goal is identifying that goal. No one can set goals for another person. For personal goal setting, individuals must know what they want, but that is only the first step in getting what they want. There is an old Chinese proverb that says, "A man can stare at a map for several years but gets no closer to his destination until he starts walking in that direction."

People should try to avoid any kind of false security that somehow, something magical happens when they set goals. Although most people who are considered high achievers would probably say that they have goals, more than likely their achievements result from focusing on their goals rather than from just setting them. On the other end of the scale, there are plenty of people with personal goals who never attain those goals.

Five hundred years ago, humans had found a way to travel across oceans by putting a large sail over a floating object. When the wind blew, everything moved in that direction. One day, however, some sailors came across an iceberg that was floating toward them. This sight totally contradicted the law of nature that they had grown to trust. How could this gigantic object be floating in a direction opposite to that of their ship and the wind? They did not understand that because 90 percent of the iceberg is submerged, it moves in the direction of the current. Herein lies the metaphor that explains the difference between goal setting and empowerment. All of the "get it done fast, make it happen yesterday," fast food to success culture wants us to think we are the sailing ship. Plot your coarse and set your sails. Be the captain of your own destiny. Unfortunately, we think like the sailboat but move like the iceberg. We are creatures of habit. Just like 90 percent of that iceberg is under the water being directed by the current, 90 percent of our behavior is being directed by our attitudes and habits.

MODEL OF EMPOWERMENT

For empowerment to take place, goals, attitudes, and habits must complement each other. In the model shown in Figure 8–1, Block One, Goals, represents the development of the blueprint. Block One starts the process in motion. It takes time to sort out current circumstances and make decisions about future goals and ways to achieve them in a relatively short period of time. Block Two, Attitudes, is a critical area because the efforts designed in Blocks One and Three need to have the support of the proper attitudes to emotionally support action. The right attitude can reduce stress as the necessary action is taken toward realizing one's goals and dreams. Block Three, Habits, is the foundation of empowerment. People are to habits, as machines are to momentum. Success is acquired through habit. People form habits, and habits form futures. A failure to form good habits deliberately may lead to the formation of bad ones unconsciously. People are who they are today because they have formed the habit of being that person. The only way to change is through habit.

Goals	Attitudes	Habits

Figure 8–1 Three-block model of empowerment. *Source:* Copyright © Achievement Dynamics Institute, Inc.

Attitudes and habits are not generally very responsive to new ideas and behavior patterns. It takes time for people to stretch these aspects of themselves until they are "synergized" with the blueprint created in Block One. It takes a while to change the "current." If the current is not flowing in the right direction, it does not really matter which way the wind is blowing. The wind is the desired outcome, but the current is reality. People will accomplish that goal when they actually develop the personal characteristics (i.e., attitudes, habits, and beliefs) to support that reality.

The tools and methods needed to direct attitudes and habits are available in Chapter 10, The Personal Empowerment Process. Also, see the model in Figure 8–2.

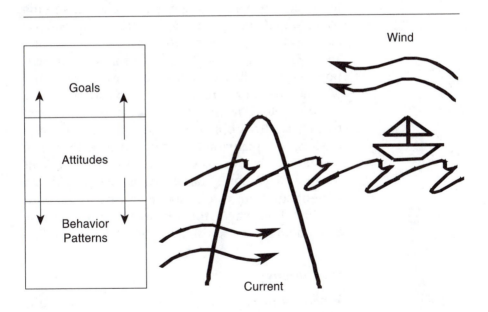

Figure 8–2 People might like to think that they can just "set their sails" for success. The reality is that they are more like the iceberg than the sailboat. What is necessary is to change the current (attitudes and habits) to move in the direction of their goals.

EXPECTATIONS OF OTHERS

People can find it very frustrating when others try to live their lives vicariously through them. The pressures that are sometimes put upon them to perform at a certain level, or in a certain area of achievement, can squeeze the enjoyment out of life. Pursuing the goals and expectations of others can temper the excitement and passion that is sometimes needed to overcome whatever obstacles may stand in the way. Commitment may falter, self-image may change adversely, and the whole experience may produce a sense of failure rather than a sense of accomplishment.

Another problem may be well-meaning loved ones who do not want to see their relatives "get their hopes up." These naysayers have made it their purpose in life to stop people from getting hurt by attempting something that may fail. Their motto is, "Take no risk and play it safe. Just be grateful for what you have and keep your nose clean." To a person seeking self-improvement, these dream stealers are like kryptonite was to Superman, zapping energy and strength. The safest way to deal with these folks is to simply keep them away from opportunity to squelch hopes and dreams. It is inadvisable to share ideas with people who are known to do this. This might be difficult because they may be family members—usually the same group from whom one might expect support. The best thing may be to wait until one's dreams have taken hold before exposing them to this cannon fire.

Dependency

Dependency means abnormal reliance on someone or something else for support. Many times people wait and hope that someone else has the answers to their problems, the money to back them, the courage to take the risk, or the know-how to make it happen. Sometimes they feel incomplete or unable to go it alone. They look for some kind of partner for the journey into the Promised Land of their plans and imagination.

It is smart to ask for help, guidance, support, and encouragement. Guidance and support can be the foundation and stabilizing force in transitions. However, everything has a hidden price tag. For example, some grown men who take over their father's successful businesses feel that their whole life has been a lie. They are often the ones with the nice cars and stylish clothes. They were the envy of all their friends through high school and college. They always seemed to have it together, entering their father's business, a very safe and protected position. They looked successful and came across as being self-assured. But the thought of carrying the responsibilities of the business on their shoulders overwhelms them, for they never developed the mental and emotional muscle needed to take on such tasks. Dealing with difficulties head on and overcoming them builds the character and confidence that are needed to take on the next set of challenges.

Partnerships

When individuals come up with exciting possibilities for their future, it can be very tempting for them to hedge their bets by soliciting partners. They may try selling their dream to someone else in hopes of developing a team effort. On the surface, it may seem like a fantastic idea, but sometimes it is born of a subconscious fear of going it alone. The key is not to allow a partnership to be an unhealthy crutch or a future excuse for failure.

A business partnership can bring a great deal of talents and abilities to a business venture. It may mean the difference between success and failure. Caution is essential in forming this kind of relationship, however. When they work, business partnerships can be as wonderful as a happy marriage; when they fail, they can be as messy as a nasty divorce. It is imperative to have a detailed business agreement, signed by both parties, one that clearly spells out each partner's contributions, obligations, and responsibilities. Some lifelong friendships are destroyed forever. The time, energy, and money that could be lost cannot compare to the damage that a partnership can cause to the relationship of people who started out the venture with a genuine love and respect for each other.

Corporate Dependence

Following total dependence on their parents as babies, as well as the safe and controlled environment of school, it is no wonder that people tend to look for a "good company" to settle into when it is time to enter the work force. The employment expectation "You do a good job, we'll take care of you" is no longer reality. Many consultants are suggesting moving away from dependent relationships between employer and employee to a more collaborative arrangement—a self-reliant model in which both parties are equal: The company needs the person as much as the person needs the company, although the arrangement may be only temporary. Individuals must ask themselves,

- Where is my security and my identity?
- Is my security of who I am only as secure as my job title?

- Do I believe that I am worth only what that company is willing to pay me at the end of the week?
- How do I define myself?
- What are my choices?
- Am I keeping my options open?
- Am I constantly creating options?
- Am I seeking out new opportunities?

The greatest asset that people have is not a job; it is themselves. The empowerment process will enable them to strengthen every aspect of their life and of who they are. They are the commodity to be shared, shined, strengthened, and enhanced.

HOME-BASED BUSINESSES

With the availability of technology and the high cost of office space, a home-based business is the envy of entrepreneurs. Minimum overhead, tax deductions on parts of the home, and no traffic hassles are some of the benefits that make a home-based business worth considering. The only challenge is, the owner of a home-based business must be self-motivated and disciplined enough to do the work at home. A home office offers countless distractions: children, chores, a favorite daytime television show, and so on. Good planning and time management are imperative.

CONCLUSION

True motivation comes from having clear expectations of what one wants from life, along with having the belief that it *can* be realized. The commitment to obtain this quality of life must be accompanied by

Notes

Notes

becoming a person who can create and support the results. A continuous evolution of goals, attitudes, and behavior patterns must occur until the person gets the right combination to break through the next success barrier.

9

The Force of Crystallized Thinking

A BLUEPRINT FOR SELF-ACTUALIZATION

Written thought is the driving force of personal motivation, goal clarification, and self-realization. The force behind it has the power to move mountains in people's lives. Through written thought, self-knowledge and self-image are defined and developed. This creates the blueprint for self-actualization.

One of the most common reasons that people stagnate in their lives is that they feel overwhelmed. They feel that they have to move as fast as they can just to keep up. They become reactive to all the demands in life and very rarely take a proactive stance on anything. Crystallizing their lives and their thoughts gives them the ability to see the big picture and respond appropriately. It helps to tap into the *moral intelligence* that lies within everyone to dive deeply into the abundance of education, training, and experience accumulated over a lifetime. Written thought forces people to be creative and cultivate solutions for the obstacles that may stand in the way of personal self-fulfillment.

It is said that "Wisdom is the balance between contemplation and action." Crystallized thinking propels people to contemplate their life. The conscious

163

awareness it brings to their moral intelligence creates a constructive discontent with the status quo. This, in turn, creates a movement of the internal "comfort zone."

FOUR LEVELS OF AWARENESS

In order to determine a person's level of awareness, it is helpful to ask the following questions:

	Yes	No
• Do you have dreams?	_____	_____
• Do you have goals?	_____	_____
• Do you have values?	_____	_____
• Do you have priorities?	_____	_____
• Do you have strengths?	_____	_____
• Do you have weaknesses?	_____	_____

If a person checked "Yes" to most of these questions, what are the top five goals in the person's life this year? In what priority are these goals? What personal values do they reflect? On what strengths does the person hope to capitalize? What weaknesses must the person overcome? What are the person's plans and objectives to bring these goals into reality? Can the person consciously explain his or her answers to these questions? If not, then the person is at level one, *"unconsciously unaware"* (Exhibit 9–1). Despite the basic knowledge of these ideas, the inability to explain them in any detail exposes a lack of conscious awareness, which, in turn, implies a lack of focus. The person who cannot focus on goals will have a very difficult time achieving them. Too many people are wondering about generalities, not about meaningful specifics.

In the second level, the "consciously unaware" level, decisions are more intuitive and introspective

Exhibit 9–1 Four Levels of Awareness

Level One—Unconsciously Unaware

You don't know that you don't know your goals, values, priorities, and that you really have no clear plan.

Level Two—Consciously Unaware

By not being able to verbally explain it, or physically write it, you now know you don't know it. The scary part is, if you don't know these things about yourself, no one else does, either. It is your responsibility to make these decisions about your life, if it is going to get done. Remember, no one knows what you want better than you—no one will be sorrier than you if you don't get it.

Level Three—Consciously Aware

Now you know what you want, why you want it, and how you are going to get it. It takes some time to contemplate these things about yourself and your life. Remember, wisdom is the balance between contemplation and action. You have imparted wisdom about yourself which took time and patience. It is your true self slowly being identified.

Level Four—Unconsciously Consciously Aware

Mental effectiveness is about reaching the fourth level of awareness and becoming unconsciously consciously aware. Real achievers make their decisions about their life on a conscious level, then turn their comfort zone of habits and thoughts over to their subconscious behavior patterns, where competency occurs naturally, free-flowingly, spontaneously, and consistently.

Source: Copyright © Achievement Dynamics Institute, Inc.

than objective. People now realize that they cannot really explain who they are or what their goals are. Those who think that they make life decisions objectively should look at the reality of the situation. What teacher would ever believe a student knew the answers for a test when he or she could not write them down? The student would not be considered "consciously aware" of it. Therefore, if people cannot write down their goals, then they do not truly know them.

People need to become "consciously aware" of who they are, what they want, why they want it, and how they plan to get it. They need to take the time to sit down and write it out, explain it, prioritize it, plan it, go back to it, and memorize it. Only then will they have the means to become "unconsciously consciously aware." The fourth level of awareness, the behavior that creates quality in life, becomes natural and automatic.

Most actions are subconscious. People operate in patterns. For example, as people get in their car and drive to work every day, the subconscious mind sends a message to the conscious mind. It says, "You can relax and think about something else during this ride. I know the way to work. I will get you there safely." So, during this ride, the driver's mind wanders on all kinds of ideas. He or she may be thinking about any number of things, past, present, and future. The one thing the driver is not thinking about is how to get to work. Further, when arriving at work, the driver is unlikely to be able to answer many questions about any details of the journey, such as whether that traffic light down the road was green or red, or what the color was of the car in front at the light. Chances are, the driver unconsciously consciously drove to work. When the route was unfamiliar, the driver had to figure out the best route. After a while, however, it becomes automatic. The conscious mind stood by only in case of emergencies, but for the most part, it was not actually involved.

Continuing this example a little further, one morning a coworker who lives nearby asks for a ride to work. On the way to work, the coworker points out a turn at an inconspicuous point that saves some driving time. Until then, the driver was unaware of this turn. The next day, when going to work alone, the driver is likely to cruise right past it as usual. Awareness of the turn changes the driver's perspective. Every day the driver becomes more determined to remember to take the new turn, until finally the driver takes it. Each day, it becomes easier and easier to remember the turn. It is only a matter of time before the new way to get to work becomes the new pattern, erasing the old way as a pattern. This is the world of behavior modification. This is the world of personal empowerment.

People find themselves in patterns in every minute of every day of their lives. They manifest this principle in managing their time, communicating, eating, and exercising. The question is, how many of these patterns have these individuals proactively developed, and how many of these patterns have they reactively developed? The key to personal empowerment is the ability to direct these patterns.

ADVANTAGES OF CRYSTALLIZED THINKING

By crystallizing information about themselves and creating clear models of their expectations, people can see more clearly the turns in the road (Exhibit 9–2). Most people want to support what they have created. The new images hold more truths about them and about their goals. When they miss the opportunity to take a new turn, a little alarm goes off to tell them that they are not being true to themselves. It is a movement of their internal comfort zone. To get comfortable again, they need to start taking the turn. This feeling can be called constructive discontent, as illustrated in the following example.

Exhibit 9–2 Why Crystallize Your Thinking

> ### *It forces you to use your imagination to . . .*
>
> - Create a solid positive image of your model self-concept and the model of your goals to be reached.
> - Challenge you to draw upon your lifetime of education, training, and experience.
> - Keep you focused on solutions, not problems.
> - Present a sense of control over situations to reduce stress.
> - Increase positive creative thinking, brainstorming, and team building.
> - Be able to work on priorities more consistently, using time more effectively.
> - Enable you to make more positive and timely decisions.
> - Develop blueprints for increasing concentration and follow-through.
> - More easily separate self from situations.
> - Increase energy levels by focusing on goals and opportunities.
> - Choose attitudes that will guarantee success.
> - Create the ability to look at the big picture, to keep things in perspective.
> - Build desire, self-confidence, and determination.
> - Become more proactive instead of reactive in your actions.
>
> *Source:* Copyright © Achievement Dynamics Institute, Inc.

Eileen was a nurse manager with a very demanding career. She was also the mother of two young children, a girl, age seven years, and a boy, age five years. As Eileen was developing the focus areas of her life, it became quite obvious that her children were a top priority. She crystallized her relationship with her children, and she decided that during the work week, her children deserved a minimum of two hours each day of quality time. She also crystallized exactly what quality time meant. It was not rushing them in the morning to day care or school, supervising their play with friends while she prepared dinner, or making sure that they took their bath and were ready for school the next day. She made a list of quality activities that allowed each child to know he or she was important and special. Some of the activities were sharing stories, talking about their day, reading their favorite book together, and doing an arts and crafts project.

At the end of the second week, Eileen was depressed. For two weeks in a row, she had failed to reach her 10 hour per week goal. Week One was six hours and Week Two was seven. As a mother, she felt that she was letting her children down. She felt that she was spending *more* time with her children now than she was before she started to monitor her activity, but *less* than she had decided was needed for her children's mental and emotional well-being.

The negative feelings that Eileen was experiencing were actually signs of progress. These feelings of inadequacy were *constructive discontent*. Before she took the time to crystallize her relationship with her children, she was doing only the minimum requirement without even realizing it. She had become painfully aware of the "turn in the road." She was aware that she was missing it. The old pattern had become unacceptable. Her comfort zone had made a drastic detour. She was available to her children emotionally, but she had not completely figured out how to fulfill this newly required level of activity. All she needed was to keep working toward finding ways to meet this goal. Her *moral intelligence* had prompted her into behavior change.

At first, Eileen's new activity level with her children would have to be a conscious effort. It is only a matter of time before new behavior patterns become natural and automatic, however. Eventually, she did reach that new level of quality time, and it became an ongoing habit. It was part of her becoming *unconsciously consciously aware* and improving the quality of life for herself and her children.

Enhancement of Critical Thinking

Just as it is difficult to add two random four-digit numbers, a basic arithmetic function, without pencil and paper, it is difficult for individuals to imagine all the complex areas of their life: (1) to identify all their values and priorities in those areas; (2) to name their goals and plans in each of the areas, and target dates for action steps; and (3) to identify and modify weaknesses along the way. The complexity of these tasks makes clear the value of a Personal Action Planner, the personal journal used for developing goals and plans. A life blueprint can identify, sort, and systematically help to modify each and every area of life.

Promotion of Mental Incubation

Those who are systematically sorting out their life in the Personal Action Planner may come across writer's block, similar to the block sometimes encountered by a novelist. It may be very difficult at times to complete a thought or an idea. When this occurs, the person should just put the Planner down and walk away. A natural process known as *mental incubation* will occur. Mentally, on a subconscious level, the person is still sorting through many possibilities and solutions. Answers or solutions may strike at any time. Experiencing success with this process will increase a person's confidence in his or her ability to think creatively through a situation. The subconscious mind is amazingly reliable in coming up with results-oriented life solutions. This is one of the best ways to tap that powerful natural resource: the power of the subconscious mind.

Creation of Time Perspective

One of the most powerful internal motivators is called *time perspective*, which is the ability to make the appropriate choices within an alignment of goals, in accordance with what is to be accomplished in the future. The further into the future that a person can visualize results, the more powerful the inclination to do the right thing today.

The further into the future people plan their financial goals, the more financially secure they become. A person with a 10-year plan rises higher on the socioeconomic ladder than a person with a 5-year plan. On the other end of the spectrum, there are the homeless who have no financial security; their time perspective is hour to hour or, possibly, minute to minute. One of the reasons that mental or physical addictions are devastating can be explained in terms of the fact that the time perspective is reduced to whenever the next "fix" may be. Here's an example: Imagine purchasing a car that will need to last a long time. What kind of maintenance program should be followed? Was the car driven like it was meant to last forever? Now, imagine leasing a car for 24 or 36 months. Would the maintenance program be any different? Would the oil be changed less frequently? Would it be driven any less gingerly? Taking it one step further: Imagine renting a car for a weekend or a short vacation. How would that car be driven? Maybe a few "Indy 500" starts, with many brake-on-a-dime stops. The point is that people are more careful, and their behavior and attitudes are more supportive, when they realize the need to extend the life of the car.

In order to take better care of themselves physically, to eat healthier food, and to exercise more regularly, people should crystallize their thinking to living to be 100. They should crystallize it, write it out, lock it in, see it, get a vision, and come up with a plan.

TECHNIQUES FOR CRYSTALLIZED THINKING

A broad variety of techniques are available for crystallized thinking.

Reverse Thinking

In reverse thinking, the person picks a point in the future, chooses an area of life, defines a goal, and finally describes that goal with all of its benefits to everyone, including the community. The vision should be made crystal clear. Then, the person considers what it would take to make that vision a reality. The steps are reversed to connect with the present.

Mind Mapping

The person who is doing a mind mapping exercise begins at the present moment and then writes all the possibilities for the next step to the goal. Adding to the puzzle of ideas, the person examines all the possibilities that would move the idea forward. The person then takes the idea in any or all directions, as determined by the thought process.

Master Mind Group

It is always powerful to bring people of like minds together for brainstorming. Carnegie felt that a master mind group was one of the great secrets of success.

He defined a master mind group as "a coordination of
knowledge and effort, in a spirit of harmony, between
two or more people, for the attainment of a definite
purpose." The energy that can be derived from such a
process is enormous. The following are brainstorming guidelines:

Notes

1. Have a clearly stated purpose.
2. If more than one person is involved, each person takes a turn, in sequence.
3. Share only one thought at a time.
4. Do not criticize each other's ideas.
5. Do not discuss each other's ideas.
6. The farther from the norm an idea is, the better.
7. It is the quantity of ideas that counts, not the
   quality.
8. If possible, build on the ideas of others.
9. It is all right to pass up a turn, if no thought
   comes to mind.
10. Make sure all ideas are recorded where everyone
    can see them.

What most often happens during this exercise is
the realization that by taking the steps needed to
accomplish a goal, even if the goal is not achieved as
expected at first, improvements will occur in the long
run.

CONCLUSION

When people take the time to crystallize their
thoughts, it becomes much easier to appeal to their
logic and creativity for decision making. They are not
so vulnerable to the fear of the unknown and do not
make decisions driven by the mercy of their emotions. Crystallized thinking is self-communication.

The contemplation needed to produce written thought enables people to tap the unlimited resources of experiences, education, training, and imagination. It enables them to use their intelligence against challenges and needs. By sorting out and thinking through a situation before time, effort, or money is invested, goals can be approached with focus, enthusiasm, and confidence.

10

The Personal Empowerment Process

The personal empowerment process is designed to enable an individual to take a step-by-step approach to self-improvement. Exhibit 10–1 illustrates the process.

Step I—*Create the Ideal Model*—In as much detail as possible, write out what is desired to be achieved. Identify present values and priorities to complement this ideal model.

A model is a person or thing considered a standard to be imitated. Once the focus areas of life have been clarified, there are several ways to create a model for the standard to enhance the quality of life.

THE POWER OF PROJECTION

The personal empowerment process utilizes the power of projection. Projection is the process of crystallizing ideas, situations, and results using mental imagery and tapping into personal resources of education, training, and experience. Several tools are available to help with the personal projection proc-

Exhibit 10–1 The Personal Empowerment Process

I. **Create the Ideal Model**
In as much detail as possible, write out the desired end results you want to achieve. Identify present values and priorities which complement this ideal model.

II. **Evaluate the Present Situation**
Evaluate the present situation in comparison to this ideal model. Identify and list current strengths and weaknesses. Maximizing strengths and modifying weaknesses is the key to utilizing untapped potential.

III. **Target Action**
Develop a practical plan with specific target dates to meet your objectives. Focus your activities toward these results. Positive results are achieved by focused action.

IV. **Generate the Right Attitudes**
Create a positive attitude about the activities that will move you to results. Your actions must become natural and automatic. Make success as much a part of the journey as the destination.

V. **Make the Necessary Commitments**
With courage and determination, recommit yourself to your goals daily, weekly, and monthly. Goals are rarely achieved with a single commitment. Every day is an opportunity to move forward more intelligently with renewed enthusiasm and determination.

Source: Copyright © Achievement Dynamics Institute, Inc.

ess. Each tool takes a combination of education, training, and experience; imagination; and personal values to establish the model that best represents each unique person.

Thinking in terms of solutions is a positive way to achieve results. People tend to live their lives in a box—a series of beliefs, patterns, and results that occur over and over again, such as diet, level of exercise, communication patterns, and ways of time management. Applying projection means concentrating, not on what it is necessary to *stop doing*, but focusing on what it is necessary to *start doing*. This is the foundation of *cognitive restructuring*. Its purpose is to focus on direction, not existence.

INCREASED LEVELS OF ENERGY

Thoughts affect a person's level of energy. At one extreme, for example, people who experience depression also lack energy. When problems arise that need to be resolved, how people approach the thinking process can affect the level of energy that people have to work on the problem. If they just ruminate over all the negative consequences of the problem, they are going to have a great deal less energy to solve it than if they cultivate all the possible solutions. Both approaches use the imagination. Despite legitimate concerns in certain aspects of life, running a negative video through the mind only causes stress and drains all hope. It is too easy to just criticize or worry about what is wrong. People need to choose to work toward solutions.

The other extreme is evident in the energy level of children as Christmas approaches. The positive expectations of Christmas day peak on Christmas Eve. Positive energy projects from people who have positive visions and expectations as to where they are going and crystallized plans to get there. Adults have a responsibility to keep creating an attitude of Christmas Eve in life, to approach life with the childlike anticipation of great things to come.

PERCEPTUAL SET

The ability of the subconscious mind to recognize and attract ideas and opportunities in the daily routine is a perceptual set. For example, a person who buys a new car, regardless of its make, model, or year, starts to notice all the other cars that look like the new car. When a woman becomes pregnant, her world is suddenly filled with maternity clothes, other expectant mothers, and newborn babies. What people perceive for themselves, they attract to themselves. Thoughts have the potential of creating their physical equivalent. Just as art imitates life, reality imitates perception. That is why some people seem always to attract opportunity, while others manage always to attract crisis.

For example, a young woman named Lillian worked as a cashier in a large supermarket. She stated her most important goal in the next two years as: "I would like to find a great guy, develop a wonderful relationship, and get married. I have really wanted this to happen for several years now, but all I do is attract jerks. If there is a jerk within 20 miles, I end up dating him, and I am tired of it. I always end up with the jerk!"

Lillian's perceptions were definitely focused on her worst fears. She was asked to build the model of her ideal mate: "Crystallize him in as much detail as possible. Write out the standards and values you see in your ideal relationship. Visualize the person and this relationship, until it is crystal clear in your mind what you are expecting to find."

Within three weeks, Lillian had a date with the bread delivery man at her job. He had been delivering there for years, but it never occurred to either of them to date. Maybe he winked at her before, and she thought it was a twitch; maybe he twitched one day, and she now mistook it as a wink. Who knows? At last report, they had married and started a family.

FOCUS AREAS

Until people have some idea as to what they want from life, they will have a difficult time identifying those goals that will bring them maximum satisfaction and self-fulfillment. As people reach new levels of success, the area of life that is being concentrated on becomes more and more focused. As part of the personal empowerment process, people choose one focus area, then imagine what life would be like if that particular area were ideal. This ideal vision would be completely satisfying, and the quality of life would be exactly as desired. This vision should be written in as much detail as possible (Exhibit 10–2). This process is good for stretching the imagination and clarifying needs and desires.

People should also mull over each focus area and decide which priorities are most important in relationship to their vision for that area (Exhibit 10–3). Obviously, some activities weigh more heavily than others.

One man who was part of a close-knit family felt that it was a priority to spend two weeks of quality time together each summer at the Jersey shore. The expense was a stretch on the family's budget, but they scrimped and saved throughout the year. There were many opportunities to spend the money elsewhere, but they felt that this time together was a real priority and well worth the effort because it reflected their goals and values as a family.

A nurse who was looking for a financial career advancement was offered a higher paying job in

---

Exhibit 10–2 Vision Model

Focus Area: Fitness and Health   Date _____

Ideal Model: 1. Going to the gym at least three times each week.
           2. Eating a balanced, low-fat, healthy diet.
           3. Weighing 140 pounds.
           4. Taking all the proper vitamins.
           5. Getting plenty of rest.
           6. Having a 32-inch waist.
           7. Body fat of 15 percent.
           8. Getting a complete checkup once a year.
           9. Having a personal trainer.

Exhibit 10–3 Personal Priority Model

Focus Area: Family   Date _____

Priorities: 1. Take a vacation together at least once a year.
              2. Have dinner together at least five times a week.
              3. Have family fun night once a week.
              4. Once a month, get the family together for a goal setting
                 meeting, where everyone discusses what their goals are for
                 that month and how everyone can help each other.

another state, but it meant uprooting her family, including two teenagers in high school. She felt it was a great opportunity, but the priority of her family outweighed the opportunity.

The values that people choose to live by set the standard for their decisions and behaviors. Others can influence personal values but cannot determine them. Only by personal reflection can people really decide what standards to live by, based on their own criteria for life decisions and opportunities. In each focus area, people must establish values as the foundation of quality results in that area of life (Exhibit 10–4).

SUNRISE VS. SUNSET

As people mature, their values change. Thus, they must continue to clarify those values. Psychologists

Exhibit 10–4 Ideal Values Model

Focus Area: My Children   Date _____

1. Always consider their well-being in all my decisions.
2. Spend quality time on a scheduled basis.
3. Be aware of how they might be feeling about things.
4. Have a relationship built on trust.
5. Always speak to them in a respectful manner.
6. Keep reinforcing a positive self-image.

have found that most people go through a revelation in their life between the ages of 35 and 45 years. When young, they tend to value quantity and external appearance. Bigger, faster, and flashier mean success. As people mature, however, they begin to equate success with quality rather than quantity and to value internal emotional satisfaction over external esthetics. The important thing to remember is that they must allow themselves to let go of outdated beliefs, values, standards, and expectations. The process is very similar to adolescence, the transition between childhood and adulthood, in that it often involves insecurities, mood swings, indecision, and a search for identity.

The emotional roller coaster of midlife is the contradiction of the goals that people have established and accomplished for themselves, because the original goals may not be compatible with the values that developed during the time it took to accomplish those goals. People also change physiologically. Obviously, 40-year-olds cannot approach their health in the same manner as 20-year-olds do. Those who do not take the time to reevaluate themselves physically, mentally, or spiritually may end up paying the price for this neglect in the long run.

MINIMUM REQUIREMENTS VS. MAXIMUM EFFORT

A habit many people learn at a young age is to look for the minimum requirements for a given responsibility. By the time they reach the fifth grade, they are experts. A teacher assigns a composition; no sooner are the topic and the due date stated, than all the hands go up to ask, "How many words does it have to be?" The students figure that it is a smart idea to establish the minimum requirements. This habit becomes a "stealth thinking process."

Too often, people make their life decisions based on the minimum requirements needed for the task. It becomes such a part of their nature that they do not even realize that they are doing it and, therefore, cannot consider its impact on their lives. They cheat themselves of the quality that they deserve in areas of life, because they do the minimum to get by. This approach drastically affects the quality of life. When the minimum people must do, becomes the maximum they are willing to do, the sum of the results is mediocrity. In addition, an opportunity for growth is lost.

Creating the ideal model and making it a part of conscious awareness makes people feel internally compelled to support what they have established for themselves. The conscious awareness is there, and comfort zones start to get uncomfortable. This feeling is called "constructive discontent" (see Chapter 9). Constructive discontent is the seed of burning desire. It is burning desire that blasts people out of complacency and into action.

CONCLUSION

Something intrinsic happens once people take the time to crystallize ideal models from life experiences, creative imagination, and personal values. These models reflect a person's innermost thoughts and being. In a very real way, each model is a vehicle for self-communication, a model of the true self. The "perceptual set" can start attracting to people the things that they see for themselves. The "constructive discontent" can start to move the comfort zones in their minds and emotions. They can begin to qualify their actions based on the "ideal models," not the "minimum requirements."

Legend has it that a man once asked Michelangelo how he was able to chisel such majestic figures out of such unsightly hunks of marble. Michelangelo replied, "I picture the man standing in the rock. Then I chisel everything away that is not the man."

Step II—*Evaluate the Present Situation as It Compares to the Model*—Identify and list current strengths and weaknesses as they relate to the model. Maximizing strengths and modifying weaknesses is the key to utilizing untapped potential.

DEVELOPMENT OF UNTAPPED POTENTIAL

The word *potential* means "something that can, but has not yet, come into being." When people rate themselves from 1 to 10, with 10 being best in any focus area of life, whether it be marriage, health, or the relationship with their children, they are quickly adding up strengths and weaknesses. If they rated themselves as a 7, it was their strengths that got them to that 7; it was their weaknesses that kept them from the 8, 9, or 10. To focus solely on strengths, while ignoring weaknesses, is unlikely to lead to significant progress, however. It is essential to identify and modify weaknesses. The secrets to greater achievements are hidden behind weaknesses.

Imagine, for example, that a nursing professor announces that there will be a major examination on four chapters of the nursing fundamentals textbook, that the test will be in one week, and that it will account for 60 percent of the semester grade. The students feel the pressure. Although overwhelmed with the amount of material to be covered, the students form study groups and work hard to prepare for the examination. The day of the examination comes, and everyone gets through it. At the following class, the instructor returns the tests with the corrections and reviews the correct answers to the questions. Then the professor makes a shocking announcement. The examination was not the major test that will count for the grade; it was only a dry run. The real examination will be similar to the dry run in that it will cover the same material, but it will take place in another week. After going through a series of mixed emotions, the nursing students spend the week studying the material that they did not know as well as they could have for the sample examination. When the real examination comes, they will be ready for it.

Behavioral scientists say that human beings are the only animals that have the ability to be dissatisfied with themselves. The ability to be dissatisfied is actually a very unique and special gift. It is the essence behind human achievement. The principles of progress can lie within the ability to seek and correct infirmities against the desired results. Each weakness is a signpost that says "Start here."

IDEAL SITUATION OR LEVEL OF DEVELOPMENT

It is helpful to begin identifying a *model* by writing a brief paragraph that describes the ideal situation or level of development in a specific area. With the use of imagination, the ideal situation can be created in great detail (Exhibit 10–5). In addition, it helps to list strengths and weaknesses in order to make the commitments for the necessary changes.

When given a chance to identify and modify their weak points, most people can seize the opportunity to work on those weak points. This process of identifying and modifying weaknesses can be very empowering to those who take advantage of the opportunity. Once they have the model, they can evaluate their strengths and weaknesses against it. They can hold onto the strengths and keep eliminating the weaknesses until only strengths remain. That is developing untapped potential, that is progress, that is driving change, that is empowerment!

SUBJECT OF EVALUATION

Any time people make a *model* of a result or activity that they hope to accomplish, they have something against which to evaluate their efforts. They are build-

Exhibit 10–5 Present Evaluation

Focus Area _____Health_____ Date ___April 19xx___

Ideal Situation or Level of Development

To weigh 160 lbs.

To be in good condition.

Present Strengths

I eat a low-fat diet.

I eat a balanced diet.

I take vitamins.

Present Weaknesses

I eat late at night.

I eat too fast.

I don't exercise regularly.

ing their mental and emotional muscle by pressing the model against their actions, not just good intentions. It is very similar to physical weight lifting, such as when the athletes stretch their muscles against the bar. The weight on the bar, the resistance, is what causes growth. By crystallizing their thoughts and intentions, people can evaluate their actual activity. The principle is the same, but the muscles are mental rather than physical.

Someone planning to start a weight training or fitness program should have a thorough health evaluation first. The program needs to be designed to modify and strengthen weaknesses. Those who have a sincere desire to improve the quality of their health must be willing to go through the pain of working on their weaknesses. A male athlete who lifts tremendous amounts of weight designed to build his already muscular arms and add size to his already enormous chest but does no exercises for his 44-inch waist is making very little significant progress in fitness or overall health.

How often are people caught in this trap? They work their comfort zones because that is where their strengths lie. Growth is not really happening. At best, status quo is being maintained. They are putting the hours in and the effort out so they can still feel good about themselves, but they are stuck in mediocrity.

PLEASING METHODS VS. PLEASING RESULTS

Which influence people more—pleasing methods or pleasing results? Empowerment comes from being more motivated by the desire for pleasing results. Mediocrity comes from being more influenced by the desire for pleasing methods (comfort zone behavior patterns) and settling for the results achieved from doing things as always.

A desire or great purpose is the strongest motivator. When motivated by needs, people stop their action steps as soon as the needs are met. Then they settle into complacency or mediocrity. People need to have a purpose strong enough to get them to *evaluate* what they are doing often enough to make the necessary adjustments in their actions to achieve that purpose. Having a vision or model to strive for helps implement that purpose.

MONTHLY EVALUATIONS

Once crystallized, the ideal model must be evaluated on a monthly basis (Exhibit 10–6). Creativity and persistence are required to make the necessary adjustments. It is helpful to make a list of accomplishments planned by the end of the month. This allows the use of reverse thinking: What results am I looking to obtain? What activity will get me there?

People who see progress are encouraged and gain a sense of satisfaction from their efforts. Those who look for perfection are easily discouraged and carry a sense of dissatisfaction, regardless of how much they have to be grateful for and proud of. A person who is always looking for progress will find it, as progress comes in many forms.

Exhibit 10–6 Monthly Evaluation Sheet

1. What were my *results* against last month's goals?
2. What *progress* did I make?
3. What *weaknesses* need to be addressed?
4. What should I *continue* doing?
5. What should I *stop* doing?
6. What should I *start* doing?
7. Goals for next month → *Urgent—Important—Miscellaneous*

Source: Copyright © Achievement Dynamics Institute, Inc.

It is important to experience a sense of growing, learning, progressing, and achieving in building self-esteem and self-image. This experience provides momentum and confidence. A sense of achievement builds self-esteem, and self-esteem builds achievement. That is the perpetual motion that drives empowerment.

Self-evaluation entails considering the negative as well as the positive. It means finding ways to see the silver lining in every cloud but not to cloud reality with denial and avoidance. It goes beyond finding ways to be efficient and effective. People need to press their results against a clear image of their expectations that reflects their values, priorities, goals, and ultimate vision of who they have decided they are and where they are going.

Step III—*Target Action*—Develop a practical plan with specific target dates to meet objectives. Focus activities toward these results. Positive results are achieved by focused action.

INTENTIONS VS. ACTIONS

People tend to judge others by their actions but judge themselves by their intentions. They let themselves "off the hook" too easily. Worse yet, most of the time they never put themselves "on the hook." Very rarely do they work from a written action plan, including an estimated time of a goal's completion. Most people take more time to plan their vacation than to plan the rest of the year—or maybe even the rest of their lives!

In order to embrace personal empowerment, people need to take the time and energy to make plans for their intentions. They must match their actions against what they said they were going to do. They must check off the things accomplished and determine what they did not do and why. Above all, they must establish the next set of action steps and attempt to reach the goals again. This plan puts mental weight on intentions so that they will turn into progressive results.

The Goal for Achievement Worksheet is useful in developing a road map for success (Exhibits 10–7 and 10–8).

- **Focus Area.** Choose the focus area that the goal is going to affect. The goal should add quality to this area of life.

Exhibit 10–7 Goal for Achievement Worksheet

Focus Area _____Today's Date _____
Target Date _____
Statement of Goal _____
Rewards of Achievement _____
_____
_____

Action Steps	Target Date	Completed (✔)
_____		❑
_____		❑
_____		❑
_____		❑
_____		❑
_____		❑
_____		❑
_____		❑
_____		❑

Additional action steps may be put on reverse. Some Action Steps may need their own goal sheet.

	Yes	No	Later
Is it worth the time, effort, and money to reach this goal?	____	____	____

Source: Copyright © Achievement Dynamics Institute, Inc.

Exhibit 10–8 Sample Goal for Achievement Worksheet

Today's Date: April 19xx   Target Date: December 19xx
Statement of Goal: Buy own home
How I will benefit from achieving this goal: More room for family, customize my
needs, choose my neighborhood, receive tax breaks, personal pride, build equity,
privacy, stability

Action Steps	Target Date	Completed (✔)
Save $15,000 for down payment	October 19xx	☐
Decide in what area we want to live		☑
Get a realtor we trust and like		☑
Develop a good credit rating		☑
Prequalify for a mortgage	September 19xx	☐
Sell boat and motorcycle for the cash	October 19xx	☐
Investigate several school systems	June 19xx	☐

Additional action steps may be put on reverse. Some action steps may need
their own goal sheet.

	Yes	No	Later
Is it worth the time, effort, and money to reach this goal?	X		

Source: Copyright © Achievement Dynamics Institute, Inc.

- **Today's Date.** Before providing any information about the goal, enter today's date. The date creates a benchmark to track progress.
- **Statement of Goal.** Create a mission statement for the goal and state it in the positive. The more specific the goal's mission statement, the easier it will be to focus on the end result.
- **Rewards of Achievement.** State all the benefits that will result from the accomplishment of this particular goal. These fruits of the action can be material, such as more money or a better car, or something less tangible like an increase of self-worth or a feeling of accomplishment. Don't forget to include how others you care about will also benefit from this goal.
- **Action Steps.** "Crystallize" objectives for those goals that require strategies to achieve them. Even

the simplest objects have a blueprint before they are put together (e.g., a chair, table, bookshelves). But where is the blueprint for life, which is so much more complicated and significant? These action steps will create personally designed life experiences.

As each action step is accomplished, it can be marked off on the goal sheet. Each check brings the goal closer. Many action steps are extensive enough to deserve their own worksheet. For example, if the goal is to earn an advanced nursing degree, it may require a significant amount of money. If the money is not readily available, a separate worksheet would be helpful to design a way to get it.

CREATION OF A TIMELINE FOR COMPLETION

Every goal must have a projected target date. Regardless of how long the goal might take, it is important to estimate projected target dates—not only for any action steps along the way, but also for the entire goal achievement process. Having a timeline for completion can only tighten the focus of reaching the goal and obtaining all its benefits. A good rule of thumb in distinguishing a wish from a goal is that a wish does not have a timeline, whereas a goal cannot exist without one.

COSTS OF MEETING THE GOAL

After filling out the Goal for Achievement Worksheet, people sometimes find that the achievement of a particular goal is not actually worth all the time and effort it would take to complete it. On the other hand, the sacrifices required may be more than acceptable, and they may be ready to make the goal become a reality. Regardless of whether this goal is worth working for or reasonable, it will be a decision based on current needs and priorities.

The time, money, and effort that the goal requires are its costs. The rewards of obtaining this goal are the benefits. If the benefits outweigh the costs, then the goal attainment should proceed. If the costs outweigh any potential benefits, it may be wise to consider abandoning the pursuit. If the benefits outweigh the costs, but the goal conflicts with a higher priority goal, then the goal sheet should be saved until there is a more opportune time to put this particular plan into action.

PROGRESSIVE VS. PERPETUATING ACTION STEPS

Progressive action steps build on each other. These action steps are accomplishments or activities that need to be done only once; then it is time to move on to the next step. Generally, they have one target date. That date may be adjusted if necessary. For example:

"Fitness" Progressive Action Steps

1. Join a gym
2. Get a physical
3. Find a personal trainer
4. Choose a nutrition program

"Finances" Progressive Action Steps

1. Open an investment account
2. Find a good financial advisor
3. Have portfolio reviewed
4. Find a better paying job

Perpetuating action steps lay the foundation for habits and behavior patterns that will support and strengthen this goal and focus area. As noted in Chapter 8, people are who they are today because they developed the habit of being that person. If they do not deliberately form good habits, then they may unconsciously form bad ones.

"Family" Perpetuating Action Steps

1. Read to the kids every day
2. Date night with spouse every week
3. At least one family meal together every day
4. Family goal-setting meeting once a month

"Fitness" Perpetuating Action Steps

1. Exercise three times a weak
2. Eat three to five servings of vegetables a day
3. Eat three to five servings of fruit a day
4. Take vitamins daily
5. Drink five glasses of water a day

Tools for Perpetuating Action Steps

1. Success Checklist—Three variations
   A. Vertical Checklist (Exhibit 10–9)
   B. Horizontal Checklist (Exhibit 10–10)
   C. Fill-in-the-Blank (Exhibit 10–11)

Step IV—*Generate the Right Attitudes*—Create a positive attitude toward the activities that will move toward the desired results. These actions must become natural and automatic. The journey should be as successful as the destination is hoped to be.

Attitude is "one's disposition." People need to generate the dispositions necessary to accomplish their goals. It is much easier to develop a positive attitude toward the results of the goal than the action; however, it is the action that accomplishes the goal.

Exhibit 10–9 Success Checklist—Vertical

Week of _____

Weekly Sales

I. Prospecting

___ (a) Secure a min. of 5 referrals/wk.
___ (b) Get adequate information on referrals
___ (c) Supplement referral prospecting with pre-approved letters
___ (d) Prospect Box and Binder organized
___ (e) Develop 1 Center of Influence/wk.
___ (f) Set up 1 seminar/wk.

II. Appointment Setting

___ (a) Have a specific time every day to secure appointments
___ (b) Use a proven approach
___ (c) A minimum of 100 dials/wk.
___ (d) Confirm all appointments
___ (e) Set 1 appointment/wk. with Human Resource, Charity, etc. for seminars

III. Presentation

___ (a) Know your presentation
___ (b) Control length of appointment
___ (c) Overcome usual objections with confidence
___ (d) Get referrals on each appointment
___ (e) Close effectively
___ (f) Set next service appointment with all existing clients

IV. Attitude

___ (a) Daily use of my Personal Development Program
___ (b) Plan each day positively
___ (c) Prepare phone calls with a positive mental attitude
___ (d) While on the phone, be sure to stay positive

V. Time Organization

___ (a) Each night, prepare "Urgent" and "Important" lists for the next day
___ (b) Develop weekly calendars
___ (c) Be on time for every meeting

---

continues

Exhibit 10–9 continued

Weekly Health and Fitness Checklist

I. Proper Nutrition

___ (a) Eat at least 2–3 servings of veggies/day
___ (b) Eat at least 2–3 servings of fruit a day
___ (c) Drink eight glasses of water per day
___ (d) Eat very little dairy
___ (e) Keep sugar consumption to a minimum
___ (f) Maintain a diet low in fat
___ (g) Eliminate fried foods
___ (h) No food two hours before bed
___ (i) Take my vitamins

II. Exercise

___ (a) Work out at least 3x/week for 30 mins.
___ (b) Warm up & stretch properly prior
___ (c) Allow exercise to become as important as eating and drinking
___ (d) Have continuous affirmations for fitness success

III. Attitude

___ (a) Keep focused and disciplined
___ (b) Visualize my end result of health
___ (c) Keep up my positive attitude

Source: Copyright © Achievement Dynamics Institute, Inc.

IMPORTANCE OF ATTITUDE

Swindoll said,

> Attitude is more important than fact. It is more important than the past, education, money, circumstances, failures, success, than what other people think, say, or do. It is more important than appearance, giftedness, or skill. It will make or break a business . . . a home . . . a friendship . . . an organization. Remarkably, you have a choice every day of what your attitude will be. We cannot change our inevitable. The only thing we can change

Exhibit 10–10 Success Checklist—Horizontal

Step One	Identify the Goal
Step Two	Identify the Action Steps
	High Pay-off Activities
Step Three	Choose a Time Period
Step Four	Create a Fill-in-the-Blank Sheet
	To Check Off along the Way

New Prospects
week of _____

Exercise
month of _____

Names		**Dates**			
1 _____		1 _____		11 _____	
2 _____		2 _____		12 _____	
3 _____		3 _____		13 _____	
4 _____		4 _____		14 _____	
5 _____		5 _____		15 _____	
6 _____		6 _____		16 _____	
7 _____		7 _____		17 _____	
8 _____		8 _____		18 _____	
9 _____		9 _____		19 _____	
10 _____		10 _____		20 _____	

Source: Copyright © Achievement Dynamics Institute, Inc.

is our attitude. Life is 10% what happens to us, and 90% of how we react to it.[1]

Behavior patterns are much like an airplane on automatic pilot. Once the plane is set on a certain course, it can still be steered manually; however, if the pilot lets go of the wheel, the plane will work itself right back into the original direction. When people force themselves to do things without changing their attitude along the way, it is only a matter of time before they work themselves back to their original behavior patterns.

Most times, if people work on a new behavior pattern with the proper affirmations (what they say to themselves) and visualizations (what they see for themselves), with repetition over a period of time, they can learn to enjoy the new action. For those who

Exhibit 10–11 Success Checklist—Fill-in-the-Blank

Week of _____								
Task	Mon.	Tue.	Wed.	Thu.	Fri.	Sat.	Sun.	Goal/Total
								/___
								/___
								/___
								/___
								/___
								/___
								/___

do not regularly get up early, exercise, and eat fruits and vegetables, for example, these actions may at first seem uncomfortable or even distasteful; if they work on these actions, however, they can actually begin to enjoy the behavior. Those new habits can become a natural and enjoyable part of life.

ATTITUDE OF ACCEPTANCE

There are things people do, not because they like to do them, but because the benefits outweigh the costs. Most men shave every morning, but few happily anticipate lathering up each day. They do not have to enjoy it, but when the time comes, they do it with very little griping or complaining.

What if every morning they went into the bathroom and stood in front of the mirror for 10 minutes, whining and complaining: "I just shaved yesterday. . . . The hairs are going to come back anyway. . . . I hate the thought of razor blades scraping across my skin." Then they finally shave. All that was accomplished by whining was self-inflicted misery. It would be mental self-flagellation.

This is just what people do when they choose a goal and perform the action steps with a negative attitude.

They are inflicting emotional pain that is, for the most part, unnecessary. Not only does it make the goal process not very enjoyable, but also it makes the goal much more difficult to achieve.

Comfort zones also influence attitude. Most people love little bunnies and have adverse feelings toward snakes. The thought of feeding a little baby rabbit to a big old snake is repulsive to many. It almost seems immoral. It is not a moral issue, however; it is a comfort zone issue. People who feed live rabbits and rodents to snakes in order to keep them alive are just following the rules of nature. Snake owners work from a different comfort zone, or set of attitudes, than those who would refuse to do the action. It can be said that the snake represents a goal. Feeding the snake represents an action.

In life, many people try to avoid what needs to be done to accomplish their goals (i.e., feeding the snake) and, in turn, "kill" the goal. Often, their self-confidence and hope die along with it. This is what happens to many goals. If people are not willing to adopt the attitudes required to accomplish the goal, the goal shrivels up and dies. They avoid the actions that they do not enjoy. Avoiding the tasks compromises their actions to the point of ineffectiveness.

When people share their goals, they often run a list of what they are *not* going to do—many times in the same breath. They seem to feel some moral obligation to avoid certain actions. One reason for crystallizing values in the focus areas is to distinguish comfort zones from morals. People must ask themselves, "Am I mentally ready to accept the responsibility that this goal is demanding? Are my attitudes in alignment? If not, am I willing to adjust my attitudes to make this happen in my life?"

One of the greatest days in life is when a person takes responsibility for his or her attitudes. It is emotion management. That is the day that person truly becomes empowered.

NEED FOR COMMITMENT

Many people stall as they progress toward the achievement of their goals because they set goals without first committing to carrying out the appropriate action. The goals linger somewhere between creation and completion. They are dreamed about, talked about, and sometimes even bragged about, but very little is done to see them through to completion.

For example, a client named Paul spent time at workshops talking about how committed he was to his new business venture. Week after week, month after month, he boasted and made known his goal. A report of his progress since the beginning of the year showed that his total time in productive activity amounted to only a couple days of work over several weeks, however. Paul was avoiding many necessary steps because each of these steps had a perceived risk of rejection or failure. His comfort zone included having the goal only as an identity; it did not allow for the actions that were necessary to bring the goal into a reality. This was like a man's telling everyone about his upcoming marriage when, in reality, he has not yet even asked the girl out on a date! Further, because Paul was stalled behind a goal that was not really happening, he did not see many other opportunities that could have developed.

Many times, changing an attitude is as easy as making a choice to feel or not to feel a certain way. Even during those extreme life situations that evoke fear, sadness, betrayal, or grief, attitude determines how people handle their feelings. Attitudes cannot always stop feelings, but they can keep feelings from stopping the achievement of goals. People who can get a grip on how they feel can more easily control those feelings.

THE BEHAVIOR PROCESS

Results are what we want.
Action is what it takes.
Feelings promote our actions.
Attitude projects our feelings.
Belief creates the attitudes.
Programming develops belief.

The behavior process is a change that takes place to create a different result in a person's life. The process starts with programming. How do people program the beliefs that they need? Consider toddlers—they have so much to learn about the world, and they undergo massive programming. They are experts at multisensory learning. They use as many senses as possible to internalize a new idea—they touch, taste, smell, look, and listen. They do things over and over again. Their minds are open to trying new things and experiences.

The way that people need to approach a new attitude is with an open mind. A baby has a limited past, but adults sometimes need to let go of the past. They must be in the process of creating the future by creating the beliefs and attitudes to support the existence of that future.

POWER OF AFFIRMATIONS—SELF-TALK

Attitudes are often a habit of thought. Thoughts always precede action, and action precedes results. The right thought patterns are more likely to produce the right results. Therefore, people must think in terms of the solution, not the problem. Thoughts have the potential of creating their physical equivalent, because people move in the direction of their thoughts. The minute an idea occurs, the mind creates an image. When the conscious mind becomes aware of something, the subconscious mind wants to attract it. For example, the person who wants to lose weight and swears off pizza is likely to think about pizza several times a day.

Unfortunately, in everyday language, affirmations are heard everywhere:

- It's going to be another one of those days.
- It's just no use.
- It just won't work.
- There's just no way.
- Nothing ever goes right for me.
- I'm so clumsy.
- I don't have the talent.
- I'm not creative.
- I can't seem to get organized.
- It's just my luck.
- I know I'm going to hate it.
- I can't seem to lose weight.
- I never have enough time.
- I get sick just thinking about it.
- I lose weight, then I gain it right back again.
- Another blue Monday.
- When will I ever learn.
- Sometimes I just hate myself.
- I'm just not good at that.
- I'm too shy.
- I never know what to say.
- I never get a break.
- I'm just not a salesperson.
- That's impossible.
- I always freeze up in front of a group.

Because no two things can occupy the same space at the same time (theory of displacement), the first step is to recognize negative affirmations and eliminate them

Exhibit 10–12 Twenty Characteristics of the Subconscious Mind

1. It is your total obedient servant.
2. It does all healing of the body.
3. It does not reason or question your command.
4. It will produce what you program into it.
5. It files and remembers every experience of your life.
6. It controls all functions of the body.
7. The greater your belief in it, the better and easier it works.
8. It never judges good or bad, right or wrong; it only obeys.
9. It works 24 hours a day, your entire life.
10. It can be programmed from an outside source.
11. It sends answers, sometimes through hunches.
12. It is the master mechanic of your body.
13. It is a creature of habit.
14. It is programmed by the spoken word, thoughts, and mental pictures.
15. It regulates your energy level.
16. It works much better when order and peace prevail.
17. It zeroes in on all goals or objectives.
18. It is oblivious of time and space; it does not know time. Only you know time. You set the timelines.
19. It is completely impersonal.
20. The better you understand it, the better it works.

Source: Copyright © Achievement Dynamics Institute, Inc.

from all thoughts and language. The subconscious mind will focus on and attract things as programmed (Exhibit 10–12). The mind can be compared to a bucket filled with water; the water, to thoughts. To get a self-defeating, limiting thought out of the mind, a person simply uses displacement—putting another thought in its place. Like polished stones heaped next to the bucket, new thoughts (with affirmations and visualizations) can be dropped in one by one, until negative thoughts have been displaced.

Rules for Affirmations

The following guidelines can be helpful in writing affirmations for success:

1. Include the first person pronoun, "I."

Exhibit 10–13 Sample Affirmative Reminders

I radiate strength and purpose.
I am patient with those around me.
I constantly improve the quality of my life in each focus area.
I am a great pro with super confidence.
I am a superstar in life.
I show warmth and concern to those I meet.
I have a magnetic strength when I speak.
I create a positive and loving home environment.
I help people to be fulfilled and happy.
I have an excellent, free-flowing memory with clear and easy recall.
I am a confident and effective decision maker.
I recommit to my goals until I get the results I want.
I have unlimited inner strength.
I have a relaxed and warm outward personality.
I am honest with myself and others.
I consistently plan my work.
I am proactive in my behavior patterns.
I plan ahead to get ahead.
I develop behavior patterns that complement my goals.
I use each minute before it disappears forever.
I keep productive work available for free moments.
I achieve the desired result with a minimum of time and energy.
I am well-organized in every phase of my life.
I treat problems as opportunities to grow and be creative.
When I choose to start, I choose to finish.
I have a constant flow of new and good ideas.
I possess an abundant supply of energy and draw upon it at will.
I am an excellent speaker, well-prepared and dynamic in my presentations.
I am completely at ease in front of any group.
I am easily able to relax and enjoy my free time.
I identify and modify any weaknesses I may have.
I meet people easily and enjoy each new association.
I take pride in a job well done.
I concentrate effectively on my goals and get results.
My energetic starts make me an achiever.

Source: Copyright © Achievement Dynamics Institute, Inc.

2. Write affirmations in the present tense.
3. State them positively.
4. Keep them realistic and specific.

After choosing the affirmations to work with (Exhibit 10–13), people can place them on separate index cards and display them in spots they see every day, like the bathroom mirror or car dashboard. It is also helpful to say them aloud as often as possible or to put them on audiotape and listen to them at least once a day.

Targets for Visualization

People should take time every day to visualize the way they want their life to go. They should see and feel it completed. They should allow their mind to rehearse procedures and events until they are clear and comfortable. Some suggestions follow:

- Mentally rehearse the day before getting up.
- Mentally rehearse working through complicated procedures.
- Mentally rehearse presentations and interviews.
- Mentally rehearse handling stressful situations in a positive, professional manner.
- Mentally rehearse for competition.
- Mentally rehearse being a winner.

ATTITUDES TO BE DEVELOPED

The purpose of this list is to identify desirable personal characteristics.

1. What actions do you presently avoid that are needed to accomplish your goals?
2. Make a list of people you admire. Then, list what characteristics you admire about each of those individuals. (This is usually a list of characteristics you would like to see in yourself.)
3. Work on strengthening beliefs you know you need to have to accomplish your life goals.

Step V—*Make the Necessary Commitments*— With courage and determination, recommit to goals daily, weekly, and monthly. Goals are

rarely achieved with a single commitment. Every day is an opportunity to move forward more intelligently with renewed enthusiasm and determination.

A *commitment* is a pledge or a promise. The moment a commitment is made, energy seems to shoot in the direction of that particular decision. Intentions are honorable, and expectations are high. What happens to that commitment?

SETBACKS

The first mistake people make when dealing with commitment is to take it too lightly. Then, they lose the personal power that commitment offers. The second most common mistake is not to recommit often enough to sustain momentum and build the circumstances needed to complete the mission.

Nothing takes the wind out of people's sails faster than realizing over a period of time that they have let themselves down. They tend to believe either that they had the wrong goal or that they were the wrong person to achieve it. They look for reasons or excuses that enable them to *not* follow through with their commitment. This is all totally unnecessary. It is perfectly natural to lose focus and attention on a new process or behavior.

The key to commitment is recommitment. People should be able to start over often enough to stretch their behavior, awareness, characteristics, and habits. The empowerment system is a system of recommitment, progress, and continuous momentum toward worthwhile and predetermined personal goals. These commitments may come in the form of isolated accomplishments or progressive behavior patterns.

A monthly cycle of reevaluation and recommitment is an excellent idea. The more frequently people reevaluate and recommit, the faster they move along in the empowerment process. Anything past 30 days seems to move into a grey area for most people. Every first of the month is a new opportunity to identify progress, address weaknesses, and redirect efforts. Concentration levels seem to diminish if people wait any longer to adjust and refocus.

THE POWER OF COMMITMENT

The level of commitment that a mother has for her child is a wonderful illustration of real commitment. In my seminar, I give a mother who has a child around seven or eight years old the following scenario:

> You and your child decide to go out hiking together. You've traveled several miles down a deserted trail and a few miles away from any road. There is an accident; your child is injured. It is not a life-threatening injury, but it is obvious that your child cannot travel. You have to bring back help. After making your child as comfortable as possible, you assure her that you'll be back as soon as you can with whatever she needs and race back to your car to get help.
>
> At this point, I ask the participant what she would do next. For every answer she gives me, I state a reason why that idea will not work. The dialogue goes something like this:

Mom: I would run back to my car.
Mario: Your car does not start. Now what?
Mom: I flag down a motorist.

Mario: No car stops for you. Now what are you going to do?
Mom: I would stand in the middle of the road so that the driver has to stop.
Mario: No other cars come. Now what?
Mom: I go to find a phone booth.
Mario: The receiver of the phone has been ripped out of the booth. What do you do next?

After several of these responses, I ask the mother when does she say, "Forget it! I've tried my best and I give up!" She emphatically says, "Never!" I then ask her what is the percent chance of her finally bringing the needed assistance to her child. She confidently says, "100 percent!" Now that is commitment! With commitment on their side when they encounter problems, people look for a way to solve those problems. Without commitment, they look for a way out.

SHORT-TERM OBJECTIVES

People should continuously identify, redefine, and accomplish their short-term objectives. Every day, every week, and every month brings with it new beginnings and a fresh perspective. In the weekly and monthly plans, objectives should be listed according to their importance (Exhibit 10–14). The weekly objective list should be separate from the monthly list, although the daily list complements the weekly, the weekly complements the monthly, and the monthly complements the yearly lists. In sum, short-term objectives should complement long-term goals, along with a person's values and priorities in life. This part of the goal-setting process helps people keep their focus and remain positive and open to new ideas at all times.

Exhibit 10–14 Short-Term Objectives

Weekly or Monthly Objectives	**Week/Month of** _____

Source: Copyright © Achievement Dynamics Institute, Inc.

LONG-TERM GOALS

Climbing Mount Everest

Rumor has it that there is a Mount Everest Club made up of people who have made the attempt to climb that majestic mountain. After every climb, whether successful or not, the Mount Everest Club throws a banquet at a beautiful lodge at the foot of the mountain. One year, after an ill-fated expedition from which there had been no survivors, the members of the Mount Everest Club made their way to their lodge at the mountain's base. This banquet would be a solemn occasion. The survivors of both successful expeditions and more unfortunate trips up the mountain assembled to await their club president, an elderly British man who was the only survivor of one of the first recorded expeditions that tried to climb Mount Everest in the late 1930s. The president's podium stood in front of a large mural of Mount Everest. This hand painting was as tall as the ceiling and loomed over the current president as he hobbled, cane in hand, to the platform for his speech. Before he started, he turned around and stared into the huge mural, which seemed to be mocking each member who had attempted to climb the mountain. Then, with a fist raised in defiance, he shouted at the painting, "Remember this, you blasted mountain! We're growing bigger, you're not!"

The visions that people have for each area of their lives can sometimes make them feel that they are climbing Mount Everest. With each plan, attempt, and commitment, they keep stretching themselves. They stretch their knowledge, imagination, character, and faith. The many commitments of new approaches and renewed enthusiasm keep their vision alive and help move them toward their goal's actualization.

Enjoying Each Plateau

There is a misconception that success is the accomplishment of a goal. If that is the only source of satisfaction, then the goal's achievement may be a very empty process. As people climb their own personal mountain, it is not just the view at the top that is breathtaking. Every plateau, every cliff, and every valley have spectacular sights to see. Every level of achievement can give a sense of personal satisfaction. People should not overlook the opportunity to take in the view at each level of the climb. Giving themselves credit for acting with initiative and recognizing their progress makes their "climb" more enjoyable and potentially more successful. With each plateau that they reach, they feel a sense of personal gratification and excitement, reassured in the knowledge that they can climb to the next plateau of challenges.

CONCLUSION

The personal empowerment process is designed to enable an individual to take a step-by-step approach to self-improvement and self-actualization. Each step is key to enhancing results and perpetuating progress. Committing again and again to the results creates the stretching and strengthening of the mental and emotional muscles needed to support one's dreams, self-concept, and moral intelligence.

NOTE

1. As cited in J.C. Maxwell, *Developing the Leader Within You* (Nashville, TN: Thomas Nelson Publishers, 1993), 97.

11

Steps to Personal Empowerment

It is not imperative to create awareness through crystallized thinking in a structured order, like an engineer building a bridge. The effort to create awareness flows more easily if people work on any part that they feel needs to be crystallized. Thus, this approach is more akin to that of a writer creating a novel or an artist starting a painting. It is not necessary to complete each section for empowerment to take place. Every tool and principle is empowering. The more tools they use and the more steps they take, however, the more empowered people become.

The principles, the tools, and the steps of the personal empowerment process combine to form an easy-to-use system to improve the quality of life continuously (Figure 11–1).

A LIST OF DREAMS

Create a wish-and-want list of all the possibilities in your heart, mind, and soul. Do not be judgmental. Do not worry about whether these ideas are affordable or practical. Have no concern for what others may say or think. Only when people have some idea of what they

211

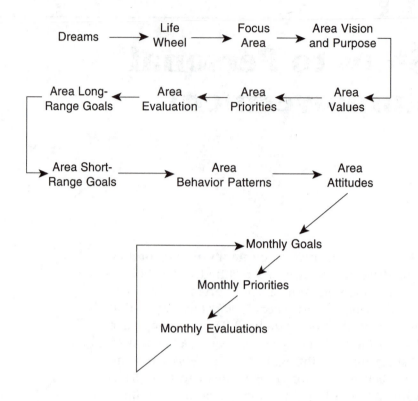

Figure 11-1 Driving personal empowerment

want from life are they able to pull together the goals that will bring the greatest enthusiasm in their pursuit and satisfaction in their attainment.

PERSONAL LIFE WHEEL

Identify the "spokes" of your life, the areas that make up your life wheel. Each of these components are referred to as your "focus area." Some examples are spouse, finances, career, fitness, home, children, recreation, and spirituality. A focus area can be anything in life that is important enough to evaluate and prioritize.

FOCUS AREA

Choose the area of your life that you think needs attention.

FOCUS AREA VISION AND PURPOSE

Create a vision and think about what your sense of purpose may be for this area of your life. Write a paragraph or make a list of how you would truly like this area of your life to look. Visualize it, and write about it in as much detail as possible.

PERSONAL VALUES

Examine the values that you choose to live by and use to set the standard for your decisions and behavior. Your values are your own, and they are a reflection of your true self.

PERSONAL PRIORITIES

Prioritize the activities and goals that are most important as they relate to your vision, purpose, and values.

FOCUS AREA EVALUATION

Take the time to look at your strengths and weaknesses in the focus areas. When you list your strengths, include everything you have to offer in this area physically, mentally, and spiritually. When you list your weaknesses, keep in mind attitudes, beliefs, and behavior patterns.

Notes

LONG-RANGE GOALS

Select what are considered "milestone dates," times of your life that are already being defined by transition, such as when your youngest child starts school or when he or she graduates from college. Possibly, a significant birthday is on the horizon. Any significant event in your future can be used as a benchmark in your life. Long-range goals could take any amount of time, from one year to the rest of your life. The tool most useful in writing out your long-range goals is the Goal for Achievement Worksheet.

SHORT-RANGE GOALS

Make a list of all the goals you would like to achieve in this focus area of your life, in the most immediate future such as 30 to 90 days. Then, do the same for the not-so-distant future in the area of three months to one year. The tools for this section could range from a daily, weekly, or monthly things-to-do list to several Goal for Achievement Worksheets.

BEHAVIOR PATTERNS

Custom-design your own behavior patterns. Habits are eventually going to make you or break you. They also change over a period of time. When healthy behavior patterns become natural and automatic, then success becomes natural and automatic. The tool best used for this process is the Success Checklist.

ATTITUDES

As you review your vision, goals, and action steps for this focus area, determine whether your attitudes and beliefs are consistent with each other. Are they congruent with your goals and plans? Make sure you are willing to fight for your goals.

MONTHLY GOALS AND PRIORITIES

Establish goals and priorities one month at a time, one week at a time, one day at a time. The more people stop to crystallize, prioritize, and reenergize, the more quickly they get to their desired destination.

MONTHLY EVALUATIONS

Navigate your way to your desired destination. Success is rarely a straight line but more like a zig-zag. It is a forward motion with many adjustments. Success is the progressive achievement of predetermined goals, worthy of your time, effort, and investments. The tool best suited for this section is the Monthly Evaluation Sheet (Exhibit 11–1).

Exhibit 11–1 Monthly Evaluation Sheet

WEEKLY or MONTHLY OBJECTIVES	WEEK / MONTH OF April 19xx
Personal:	Business:
1. Finish yard	1. 100 cold calls
2. Easter dinner at our house	2. 40 referrals
3. Build treehouse for the kids	3. 30 new appointments
4. Take Reneé out to dinner	4. Place ad in paper
5. Visit Aunt Mary	5. Finish proposal
6. Update software	6. Update mailing list
7. Change oil in both cars	7. Order new business cards
8. Work out 12 times	8. 20 new clients
9. Set up vacation with the family	

Source: © Achievement Dynamics Institute, Inc.

Notes

CONCLUSION

The steps to personal empowerment are a way to progressively identify, clarify, and, where needed, modify strengths, weaknesses, actions, and results. In order for results to take place, it is not necessary to do each step in a certain order. All of the tools present an opportunity for self-clarification and personal direction. The more people understand their true self-concept, the easier it is for them to stand their ground and plow through challenging circumstances toward success.

12

Time Management

Benjamin Franklin once said, "Time is money." In reality, however, time is much more valuable than money. If a person loses or wastes money, that person can make it again. If that person loses or wastes time, it is gone forever. It is a shrinking commodity. How and where people invest their time directly relate to the quality of life. Time management is about doing the appropriate actions when necessary in accordance with goals, values, and a sense of purpose in creating quality in life.

A college professor once used this demonstration to educate his students on the principles of time management. He placed a five-gallon glass jar on top of a laboratory bench in front of the class. From underneath the bench, he pulled up a sack of rocks and proceeded to fill the glass jar to the top with rocks. Then he asked the class, "Is this jar full?" The class responded, "Yes." He said, "Ah, but wait!" He then pulled a pitcher of gravel from underneath the bench and proceeded to dump gravel around the rocks in the jar. When he could fit no more gravel in the jar, he asked the class again, "Is this jar full?" The class, now catching on, said, "No." He said, "Right!" He then pulled a pitcher of sand from beneath the bench and poured the sand all around the gravel in the jar.

217

When he could fit no more sand in the jar, he asked the class again, "Is this jar full?" The class said, "No." He said, "Right!" He then proceeded to pull from beneath the bench a pitcher of water. He poured the water to the top of the glass jar. Then he asked the class, "What did you learn from this?" The class, discussing it, came up with a unanimous answer and said, "There is always room for more." He said, "No. We need to put the rocks in first!"

So many times people say that they do not have time for the activities that lead to quality in their life, such as exercise, quality time with their children, fun and relaxing recreational activities. However, in business, it could be those seemingly impossible activities that make you the most money. These are the "rocks" in life that must be put in first. Activities chosen as priorities in life need to be scheduled on a daily, weekly, and monthly basis. They often rest in perpetuating action steps that are part of the ongoing checklist, which is why the checklist system works so well. The renewing of the cycle and competing against oneself week after week, month after month, stretches the behavior patterns and allows the new pattern to take shape. At first, it is a real struggle to find the time. It takes an open mind, a little discipline, and a generous dose of creativity.

TIME AND BELIEF

People have an abundance of time. They have 24 hours a day, renewable every day from the day they are born to the day they die. The first step is really believing that time is abundant. If people believe that there is not enough time to do the things that add quality to their life, they will have a very difficult time finding ways to implement their high-priority activity as they operate on a day-to-day basis. These people need to find out where their time is going, to define their goals clearly, and to determine what activities, progressive and perpetuating, achieve those goals. That is the model.

The second step of the empowerment process has to do with evaluating the present situation. Implementation of a Daily Time Use Analysis may be challenging (Exhibit 12–1), but the value of the information and awareness level can be life changing. It requires individuals to track their time Monday through Friday, from the time they awaken until the time they go to bed.

At the end of each day on the Weekly Time Survey (Exhibit 12–2), they add up tasks to see how much time was spent on each task, each day. At the end of the week, they add up the total time spent on each task. Recent studies have shown that 40 percent of the average U.S. citizen's free time goes into watching television. Each person must decide if the time taken to do each task during that week is worth it. They then calculate the time:benefit ratio, which involves weighing the amount of time it takes to do a task against the benefits of doing the task.

This evaluation of time and analysis of activities is where time management begins. For those who are truly committed to finding the time needed to do the things that improve the quality of their life, this survey is crucial. It is extraordinary how quickly time moves and how rapidly time can add up. Several years ago, I analyzed my own use of time. I discovered that I was spending more than two hours each day in news-related activity: the morning show, newspapers, the evening news, and CNN. Using the time:benefit ratio, I felt that the amount of time taken from my life by this activity was not equal to, or greater than, the benefits I was receiving. I decided to read the paper only 15 minutes each day, a little longer if necessary. Calculating the time I had been spending, two hours

Exhibit 12–1 Daily Time Use Analysis

Date _____		
AM	**How I Spent My Time**	**Minutes Wasted**
6:00		
6:30		
7:00		
7:30		
8:00		
8:30		
9:00		
9:30		
10:00		
10:30		
11:00		
11:30		
PM		
12:00		
12:30		
1:00		
1:30		
2:00		
2:30		
3:00		
3:30		
4:00		
4:30		
5:00		
5:30		
6:00		
6:30		
7:00		
7:30		
8:00		
8:30		
9:00		
9:30		
10:00		
10:30		
11:00		

Total Time Wasted Today _____

Source: Copyright © Achievement Dynamics Institute, Inc.

Exhibit 12–2 Weekly Time Survey

Task	Mon.	Tue.	Wed.	Thu.	Fri.	Sat.	Total
Week of _____							

Source: Copyright © Achievement Dynamics Institute, Inc.

per day times five days per week comes to 10 hours per week, or 40 hours per month, the average workweek. If accumulated over a year's time, it comes to 12 workweeks, which is three months' working full-time.

THREE Ds OF TIME MANAGEMENT

There are three Ds in time management: Disregard, Delegate, or Do It! The Time Management Sheet (Exhibit 12–3) can be useful in prioritizing time. Once people look at where their time is going, they need to look at what they can disregard and then what they can delegate. Parents often say, "I have several children, I have no time." In reality, they have several children to whom they could be delegating much of their activity, allowing for more quality time to focus on building a good relationship with their children. Then there is "Do It!" Once they decide what it is that they need to do, they can develop that activity into a habit. They need to put the rocks in first!

Exhibit 12–3 Time Management Sheet

Day/week/month _____
Urgent
_____
_____
_____
_____
Important
_____
_____
_____
_____
Miscellaneous/notes
_____
_____
_____
_____
Source: Copyright © Achievement Dynamics Institute, Inc.

CHRONOS VS. KAIROS

The linear measurement of time is called chrono-logical time, from the Greek word *chronos*. The Greeks had another way of measuring time, however. They also had the word *kairos*, from which they derived the kairological measurement of time. The growth mea-surement of time, this is the time it takes for maturity and is not always measurable in chronological terms. For example, the person who wants to grow pump-kins picks out a date in the spring to turn the soil, chooses the right time to plant the seeds, regularly waters the seeds, cultivates the ground, and weeds the garden. These are all chronological timelines. The person cannot say, "On October 15, we will pick seven 15-pound pumpkins from this pumpkin patch." It is not possible to designate chronologically when the pumpkins actually appear, their size, and quantity. This is a very helpful philosophy to keep in mind when working toward goals and developing those things that will bring quality to life.

Many times, when people start a business, it does not grow as rapidly as their projected chronological dates. This creates discouragement. The owners do not realize that, at the same time, the business is growing in a kairological sequence. They can chronologically add more activities in a shorter period of time or even heighten the quality of activities, but ultimately, kairologically, the business will develop and grow at its own pace. Many times in life, it is helpful to step back and look at growth in terms of kairological time, not chronological time.

CONCLUSION

Time is one of the most precious commodities. It is a shrinking, nonrenewable asset. People do not have the power to slow it down, nor is there any guarantee of tomorrow. The opportunity to enjoy life and bring joy to others passes all too quickly, so it is every person's responsibility to invest time wisely.

13

Finding a Life Partner: Types of Personality Evaluations*

TEMPERAMENT AWARENESS

A Temperament Awareness Profile is one of the most personally revealing evaluations we can have done. They help us identify the patterns of behavior we feel most comfortable in. Matching our "behavior type" with our work environment is an ideal way to reduce stress on the job, create enthusiasm, and increase productivity. Every person has his or her special way of doing things. It all translates into identifiable and predictable behavior types which represent the way you get things accomplished and the way you deal with people and situations.

All of the behavior type indicators are designed to help us see our predisposed patterns of behavior. However, these indicators identify tendencies not

*Information about the DiSC® model and DISC® Dimensions of Behavior is taken from the *Personal Profile System* © Copyright 1994, Carlson Learning Company, and is used with permission of Carlson Learning Company. "DiSC" and "Personal Profile System" are registered trademarks of Carlson Learning Company, Minneapolis, Minnesota. For information call 800-777-9897.

To become an authorized DiSC® personality profile trainer and distributor with the Carlson Learning Company, call Achievement Dynamics Institute, Inc., at 800-784-6257.

Notes

225

certainties. Depending upon what is needed in a particular situation, we have the ability to adapt our behavior to get the job done.

For example, if people who have a natural tendency not to be overly concerned with details find themselves faced with the responsibility of a mortgage application, they would be somewhat uncomfortable with all the minute components. But have no fear, if the desire to accomplish the task is great enough, the job could be handled quite well.

TWO MAJOR SPECTRUMS OF PERSONALITY

Two major spectrums of personality are introversion and extroversion. An introvert has a tendency to enjoy the confines of solitude. The idea of a good time for an introvert is finding a good book, a quiet room with a fireplace, and a cup of fine java. They gain energy by being alone, and lose energy by interacting with several people over a prolonged period of time. The extrovert, on the other hand, is most comfortable interacting with as many people as possible—if people aren't readily available, almost any type of warm-blooded animal will do. The extrovert seeks outside stimulation. They gain energy by being around others and lose energy by spending time alone. If a introvert and extrovert are dating and attend a party togther, after several hours, the introvert can't wait to go home to peace and quiet, while the extrovert enthusiastically calls out an open invitation for anyone who wants to stop at the diner on the way home.

In 1923, Dr. Carl Jung wrote the breakthrough book *Psychological Types*. It was the most sophisticated scientific work ever published on personality patterns at the time. Millions of dollars and many years of research have combined to create more then a dozen varied concepts on temperamental differences. The common denominator of all the variations is the act of dividing people and their behavior styles into groups. Now, using the four classifications of DiSC from the Personal Profile System,® let's explore what each of the four DiSC dimensions of temperaments has to offer. Keep in mind that people will have varying degrees of each of the four behaviors. At the end of this chapter there will be a chart for comparisons with other behavioral indicators.

The D-i-S-C in the Personal Profile System represent the four categories of behavior:

DOMINANCE — INFLUENCE — STEADINESS —
CONSCIENTIOUSNESS

HIGH-D—DOMINANCE

Dominance (High-D) individuals demonstrate aggressiveness and are competitive, decisive, and quick to take action. They respond positively to challenge and are always ready to take on (sometime usurp) both responsibility and authority. These individuals can become frustrated and bored if things become too predictable.

Strengths

- Competitive
- Decisive
- Results oriented
- Moves quickly and energetically
- Takes on responsibilities
- Can work under pressure and also apply it
- Needs to be active
- Direct and straightforward

High-D people work best for a boss whose competence they can respect. Since the High-D reacts positively to openness and honesty, it is important that the limits of authority be clearly communicated and enforced. The ideal environment has a fast track with challenging and unique assignments, plenty of opportunity to prove themselves, and the authority to see things through. The High-D tends to move up or to move on. They'll get results, but the price for those results is often change.

Potential Problem Areas

Planning	Controlling
Tends to be a fire fighter, manages by crisis	May be a poor delegator
May neglect the long range	Tends to be impatient
	Tries to do everything alone
	May instill fear

Remember, a High-D may want:

- Authority, challenges, prestige, freedom, varied activities, difficult assignment, logical approach, opportunity for advancement.
- You to provide direct answers, be brief and to the point. Stick to business.
- To be asked "What" questions, not "How." Logic of ideas or approaches stressed.
- Possibilities outlined for them to get results, solve problems, be in charge.
- When you are in agreement, agree with facts or idea, not person.
- Time lines or sanctions to be brought into the open, and related to the end result/goal.

Also known as:

1. Driver by Merrill, Wilson, Alessandra, and Hunsaker
2. Controller by DeVille
3. Choleric by Galen and Hippocrates
4. Controlling-Taking by Atkins
5. Q1 Dominant-Hostile by Lefton

HIGH-I—INFLUENCE

Influence (High-i) individuals demonstrate verbal prowess, are outgoing, and prefer working with people to working with things. People generally respond well to the High-i's natural ease and charm which is particularly fortunate, as High-i's need others to like them. While the High-i likes center stage and is good at verbalizing, he or she must be careful not to be perceived as superficial. On occasion, the High-i has been known to try to substitute charm for performance. Wanting things to run smoothly, High-i's tend to abdicate when confronted by people problems. The High-i individual may also put more stock in impressions than facts, and as a result, sacrifice thoroughness to speed.

Strengths

- Persuasive
- Optimistic
- Self-confident
- Easy to meet
- Poised
- Enthusiastic
- Good at motivating others
- Friendly and open

High-i individuals work best for a boss who will allow them to do their own thing. The High-i likes variety and freedom coupled with the opportunity to be impressive. He or she will perform best under close but not stifling supervision. The High-i is better at promoting than fact-finding motivating than interpreting and promising then delivering. Well-defined standards of performance, established deadlines, and monitored checkpoints are of great help to the High-i, although he or she may initially resist these measures. The High-i is especially good at initiating people-oriented projects (where a "sell' is required) but not always good at follow-up and follow-through. You must always listen carefully to the High-i's reason(s) for not meeting deadlines to effectively distinguish reason from rationalization.

Potential Problem Areas

Planning	Controlling
Prone to superficial analysis and generalizations	May abdicate responsibility and buy excuses
Tends to trust people more than facts	May be too trusting
May underestimate problems and overestimate results	May not detect the warning signals

Remember, a High-i may want:

- Social recognition, popularity, people to talk to, freedom of speech, freedom from control and detail, favorable working conditions, recognition of abilities, to help others, the chance to motivate people.
- A friendly environment with time for stimulation and fun activities.
- A chance for them to verbalize about ideas, people, and their intuition.
- You to provide ideas for transferring talk to action with incentives for starting tasks.
- Testimonials of experts on ideas and details in writing which are not dwelled upon.
- To be involved in democratic relationships.

Also known as:

1. Expressive by Merrill, Wilson, Alessandra, and Hunsaker

2. Entertainer by DeVille
3. Sanguine by Galen and Hippocrates
4. Adapting-Dealing by Atkins
5. Q4 Dominant-Warm by Lefton

HIGH-S—STEADINESS

Steadiness (High-S) individuals are usually calm, friendly, and low-key. Hard working, well-organized, loyal, and sincere, the High-S is a good team player, especially when he or she feels appreciated. When the High-S feels left out, however, he or she will tend to slow things down and will not demonstrate much "sense of urgency." Since High-S persons are very patient, they can be counted upon to complete tasks and detailed projects. The High-S individual is usually well-liked, is good at maintaining a so-called "open door policy," and is generally one to whom you can "tell all" without fear of being judged prematurely.

Strengths

- Reliability
- Listens well
- Well-organized
- Systematic
- Patience
- Dependability
- Finishes what is started
- Friendly

The High-S individual will work best for a friendly boss who takes a genuine interest in him or her as both a worker and as a person. High-S's work best at a self-established pace in a secure and well-structured environment. Change tends to disrupt High-S performance, because they identify with the group or organization (i.e., "My company," "My boss," "My team"). The High-S's patience and natural good listening ability tend to make him or her a "confidante" and sounding board within any organization. Because High-S persons prefer a one-task-at-a-time approach, they may not always move fast enough to suit others.

Potential Problem Areas

Planning	Controlling
May be more task oriented than concept oriented	Believes that time is the great healer
Prefers a well-defined "things to do today" approach	May be too patient for results
	Can be too meticulous
Tends not to ask for help from others	Tends to stay with the tried and true

Remember, a High-S may want:

- Status quo, security of situation, time to adjust, appreciation, identification with group, work pattern, limited territory, areas of specialization.
- A sincere, personal, and agreeable environment.
- A genuine interest in them as a person with personal assurances of support.
- To be asked "how" questions to get their opinions.
- Patience in defining their goals while emphasizing how their actions will minimize their risk.
- Ideas or departures from status quo presented in a non-threatening manner.
- Clearly defined roles or goals and their place in the plan.

Also known as:

1. Amiable by Merrill, Wilson, Alessandra, and Hunsaker
2. Supporter by DeVille

3. Phlegmatic by Galen and Hippocrates
4. Supporting-Giving by Atkins
5. Q3 Submissive-Warm by Lefton

HIGH-C—CONSCIENTIOUSNESS

Conscientiousness (High-C) individuals are accurate, attentive to detail, and disciplined and are very rarely caught unprepared. The High-C individual can be and usually is very strict — normally backing various orders with quotes from the "book," the "rules," or some other higher authority. The High-C is innately cautious, prefers avoiding trouble to confronting it, and so may appear evasive. People high in the Conscientiousness factor are good technically and tend to count on facts, details, and statistics to do their "fighting" for them. A very interesting facet of the High-C behavior is his or her sensitivity to criticism, although they are adept at finding errors of both omission and commission in the work of others.

Strengths

- Precise
- Well-prepared
- Plans thoroughly
- Checks and double checks
- Attentive to detail
- Can anticipate problems

The High-C individual will work best for a boss who does not press for results "yesterday." In addition, the High-C individual needs and wants sufficient lead time to do a complete and thorough job. They prefer an environment where accuracy is valued, along with a good measure of personal integrity on the part of superiors. The High-C individual is well-suited to assignments requiring persistence, data collection and interpretation, dealing with tasks rather than people. Regardless of the type of work, the High-C will be much more productive when everything is all neatly packaged into a system of well-defined goals, checkpoints, and accurate data.

Potential Problem Areas

Planning	**Controlling**
May plan more than do	May over-supervise, being
May concentrate on the	slow to trust others
"Small" picture	May insist on too much
Tends to move slowly and	written documentation
perhaps too cautiously	Requires you constantly
	check back in with them
	May never be satisfied

Remember, a High-C may want:

- One-on-one relationships, emphasis on accuracy, exact job description, controlled work environment, no emotional outbursts.
- You to take time to prepare your case in advance.
- Straight pros and cons of ideas. Ideas supported with accurate data.
- Reassurances that they have all the facts.
- An exact job description with precise explanation of how it best fits the big picture.
- You to: If agreeing, be specific. If disagreeing, disagree with facts, not person.
- You to be prepared to provide many explanations in a patient, persistent manner.

Also known as:

1. Analytical by Merrill, Wilson, Alessandra, and Hunsaker
2. Comprehender by DeVille
3. Melancholy by Galen and Hippocrates

4. Conserving-Holding by Atkins
5. Q2 Submissive-Hostile by Lefton

NOTES

1. Alessandra, Anthony, Ph.D., and Wexler, Phillip. *Non-Manipulative Selling* (Reston Publishing Company, 1979).

2. Atkins, Stuart, *The Name of Your Game* (Stuart Atkins, 1982).

3. Burton, Richard, *The Anatomy of Melancholy*.

4. DeVille, Jard, *Nice Guys Finish First* (William Morrow & Company, 1979).

5. Galen, Claudius, Second Century A.D. Philosopher and Physician, as referenced by Carl Jung in *Psychological Types*.

6. Carlson Learning Company, Personal Profile System,® Personal Profile System® Facilitation Kit.

7. Gorovitz, Elizabeth, *The Creative Brain II: A Revisit with Ned Hermann*.

8. Hunsaker, Phillip, Ph.D., and Alessandra, Anthony, Ph.D., *The Art of Managing People* (Spectrum, 1980).

9. Jung, Carl, *Psychological Types* (Harcourt, Brace & Company, 1924).

10. Lefton, Robert, *Effective Motivation Through Performance Appraisal* (John Wiley, Inc., 1977).

11. Merrill, David, and Reid, Roger, *Personal Styles and Effective Performance* (Chilton Book Company, 1981).

12. *Training and Development Journal*, December 1982, pp. 74–88.

13. Wilson Learning Corporation, *Social Styles Sales Strategies* (Wilson Learning Corporation, 1977).

14

Networking

One of the most important tools for people who are looking for new career and life opportunities is a willingness to open their "nets" to gather as many contacts and as much support as possible. As they move through change and transition, their lives can be made much easier if they have other people's help to generate new ideas and different possibilities. Networking helps people to look for what they want and go out and make it happen. Thus, people should widen their sphere of influence, gaining as many contacts with as many people, organizations, and opportunities as possible. Becoming a master networker can be fun and profitable. There is an energy source to be tapped.

Networking can be considered an art, a science, and a technology. It is a teachable and learnable process that anyone can master. It does take a personal commitment to develop it, do it, and stick with it. Like anything else, at first some of the ideas may seem uncomfortable, but a change in attitude can make it work.

TYPES OF NETWORKING

Master Mind Alliance. Bring together a group of positive individuals periodically for the purpose of

237

setting goals, sharing leads and information, and brainstorming solutions and possibilities. Each person will bring a unique perspective to the process of creating a network. The most important thing to remember during these regular meetings is to keep the focus toward solutions, not problems.

Previous Clients/Contacts. Make a list of all of the people, companies, organizations, and associations you have worked with in the past. Think of all the ways these contacts can help you now. Maybe there is some work you can do for them on a freelance or a private consulting basis. Who are their networks and contacts? Discuss their information with the people in your master mind group.

Friends and Relatives. Who do friends and relatives know? What ideas can they bring to the table? It is a very good idea to let them all know your situation and your intentions. You could send a general letter to all your family and friends, and then follow up with a telephone call. As with all contacts, consistent follow-up is of vital importance. Unless you follow up on a regular basis, people will unintentionally forget to keep you in mind. The key is to affect their perceptual set, to keep their subconscious mind working for your best interest.

Endless Chain of Referrals. Have completely written out all the types of people, places, and situations that interest you. Visualize it in as much detail as possible. This will make it possible for you to communicate with your contacts much more clearly and make it easier for them to help you. Every time you are referred to another person, ask that person for the same type of contacts. It is also a good idea to keep an index card for each referral with all the relevant information on the card, including the name and telephone number of the person who made the referral. You may have to recontact the referring person for more information.

Nest. Any type of existing group or association that meets on a regular basis can be called a nest. The more closely the organization is associated with the field of individuals you want to meet, obviously the better your chances are of making a connection. Professional nursing associations, especially those groups that deal with more specialized fields of nursing, can be a great source of personal support and employment opportunities. For example, local chapters of oncology nurses, enterostomal nursing, occupational health, case management, and critical care organizations can be very helpful. Attending some of their meetings will provide a feel for the group. Then get involved. Volunteer to be on one of their committees and get to know the other members. Good committees include program, membership, and hospitality. Local chapter board nominations are generally chosen from the ranks of their most active members, so it really does pay to be involved. The more often you attend these meetings, the better your networking success rate. Further, do not be too judgmental about any person or group; the best lead may come from the most unlikely source.

Centers of Influence. An individual who is respected and well connected in the community is a center of influence. One of these people can open doors fast and often. Make a list of the people who qualify. These individuals may be in positions of power, well loved, or just highly respected in the community. Whatever the reason is for valuing this person's opinion, it is vitally important to show respect and appreciation when a step is taken on your behalf.

Personal Observation. Keep your eyes and ears open. Wherever you go, be aware of all the opportunities that pass your way every day. The more you become aware of what you are looking for, the more efficient your perceptual set. Always be ready for the right person, place, or thing to pop into your grasp at any time.

Public Speaking. Earn the right to speak on something in your area of expertise. Interesting public speakers are always in demand. If you need assistance or practice, join a Toastmasters Club, or take a public speaking course. Toastmasters is world renowned, usually local and inexpensive. If the thought of public speaking scares you, just keep in mind, "Do the thing you fear and the death of fear is certain."

Volunteer Organizations. One of the best ways to meet exceptional people is through volunteer work. Look for agencies that complement your interests. Many organizations in which it is difficult to find employment opportunities have some volunteer opportunities. These organizations may hire only from personal references. Employment openings like those never appear publicly. Not only does volunteering give you added experience, but also it can assist in building contacts and relationships that enable you to break into a new field. If the type of job you want is on a public payroll or a quasi-government organization (or receiving federal, state, or county funds), consider volunteering with a local political organization.

Cold Canvass. No networking program would be complete without cold canvassing. The cold canvass methods most commonly used are direct mail and telemarketing. Both of these systems get best results when the list being used is updated and pertinent to your request. Make sure your materials are of good quality if you are using direct mail and your telephone approach is calm and sincere if you are telemarketing. It helps to write a script of the questions to ask and the explanation to give for making the call. Persistence and practice improve your skill at cold canvassing.

CONCLUSION

It is wise to use as many of these networking opportunities as possible. To get the best results, people need to set their networking goals, take the necessary action, and keep recommitting themselves to the process. Developing and cultivating an ongoing outreach of contacts and associations multiplies one's chances for opportunity and success. It is the old "it's not what you know, it's who you know" reality. Use the power of it to create a network that may open many doors for years to come.

Notes

Appendix

Glossary of Terms and Definitions

Actions/Decisions—Choices made to create an opportunity or minimize a loss.

Affirmations—Personal constructive or destructive statements that direct behavior, support beliefs, or develop attitudes.

Affirmative Reminders—Statements of fact or belief designed to prepare individuals for reaching a predetermined, worthwhile outcome or goal. A statement of the goal describing the goal setter as though his or her desired goal or attitudinal change has already been achieved.

Association—The method in which people relate to a current situation by referring back to past experiences.

Attitude Motivation—Motives for action based upon the positive well-being of an individual.

Attitudes—Beliefs, opinions, and ideas that sway an individual toward a certain course of action.

Awareness, Personal—A conscious knowledge of oneself. It is specific to goals, values, priorities, and actions.

Checklist (Horizontal and Vertical)—A personal tool used to keep track of activities leading to goal achievement. These checklists are specifically used to create new behavior patterns.

Chronos—The Greek word for linear measurement of time; chronological time.

Cognitive Restructuring—Changing a thought process to alter emotions or behavior.

Comfort Zone—Routine behavior that may prevent individuals from making the changes that would have the ability to improve the quality of their life.

Conditioned Awareness—Perceptions created by the repetition of ideas or personal experiences.

Crystallized Thinking—Well-defined written thought.

Effectiveness—The degree to which personal actions relate to the quality of an individual's life.

Evaluation—The identification of personal strengths and weaknesses for the purpose of directing change.

Fear Motivation—Motivation based on the anticipation of loss, failure, and/or embarrassment.

Focus Area—An area in life that requires and deserves attention. The quality of this area directly affects one's happiness, peace of mind, and well-being.

Identification/Modification—Proactively changing or preventing weakness.

Incentive Motivation—These goals are motives for action based upon reward. They tend to be temporary and for the short term. The reward must increase in order for the action to continue.

Kairos—The Greek word for the growth measurement of time; kairological time.

Motivation—The driving force behind an action.

Objectives—Short-term goals to be accomplished on a daily, weekly, and monthly basis.

Perception—The way the world is seen through an individual's attitudes and beliefs. This reality is not always complete or accurate.

Perceptual Set—The ability of the subconscious mind to recognize and attract ideas and opportunities into daily routines.

Personal Best—Being in competition with oneself to progressively improve focus, activity, and results.

Personal Empowerment—The ability to improve the quality of one's life through a continuous process of personal expansion, exploration, and emotional development.

Potential—The innate ability to create opportunity, overcome adversity, and contribute to humanity.

Priorities—The order in which action is taken, based upon the desired result and personal values.

Responsibility—Realizing and accepting the consequences of one's choices and actions. An equal willingness to accept accountability for faults and recognition for accomplishments and success.

Self-Esteem—The belief in one's potential and abilities.

Self-Image—How people see themselves based upon the accumulation of experiences and thought patterns.

Self-Talk—An individual's words that trigger pictures, emotions, and feelings which, in turn, can affect attitude (self-image).

Stress—An inward emotional response based upon a person's perception of the severity of an event. There is both positive stress and negative stress.

Stuck—Remaining stagnant in personal growth and results.

Success—The accomplishments achieved by a continuous process of personal expansion, exploration, and emotional development. *Success is a journey, not a destination.*

Values, Personal—The standards by which a person makes life decisions. Values are used to judge the importance of an individual's own accomplishments.

Visualization, Mental—Rehearsing an image, in the mind's eye, to be accomplished and experienced in reality.

Index

History of case management, 105–106
HMO. *See* Health maintenance
    organizations
Holistic health, 66
Home-based business, 161
Hospital beds in United States, 4

I

Identification/modification, defined, 244
Imagination, need for, 138–142
Incentive motivation, 153
    defined, 244
Influence, centers of, networking, 239
Intentions *vs.* actions, 188–191
Intermediate care, case managers, 114–115
Internal case management, 112–115
Internet, 32
Intranet, 32

K

Kairos
    vs. chronos, 222–223
    defined, 245

L

Legal risks, 20–21
Levels of awareness, 164–167
Life partner, 225–235
    High-C—consciousness, 233–235
    High-D—dominance, 227–228
    High-I—influence, 229–231
    High-S—steadiness, 231–233
    personality, major spectrums of,
        226–27
    temperament awareness, 225–226
Life wheel, personal, 136–138, 212
Linkage, 22–227
    in health care system, 22–27
    operational, 26–27
    strategic, 23–26
Long-term care, case managers, 114–115
Long-term goals, 208–209

M

Manager, business behavioral style, 98
Manual of Current Procedural
    Terminology, 12–15
Master mind alliance, 172–173, 237
Medicaid, 9–10
    hospital satisfaction, identification
        of, 24
Medicare, 7–8
    hospital satisfaction, identification
        of, 24
Mind mapping, 172
Model of empowerment, 156–57
Monthly evaluations, 187–188, 215
Monthly goals, 215
Motivate, defined, 152
Motivation, defined, 245
Motivators, external, 152–153
Myths regarding value, 10–11

N

Needs, patients presentation of, 64–65
Nest, networking and, 239
Networking, 100–101, 237–241
    centers of influence, 239
    cold canvas, 240
    contacts, 238
    friends, 238
    master mind alliance, 237
    nest, 239
    personal observation, 240
    previous clients, 238
    public speaking, 240
    referrals, endless chain of, 238
    relatives, 238
    types of, 237–241
    volunteer organizations, 240
Nonprofit, defined, 15
Nonprofit corporations, characteristics
    of, 15
Nursing skill set, matrix, 90–101

O

Objectives, defined, 245

power of, 200–204
Settings, for case management, 112–116
Skill set, training, 98–100
Skills, transferable, identification of,
86–90
Social service model, case management,
113–114
State regulators, hospital satisfaction,
identification of, 24
Stimulation, 152–53
Stress, defined, 246
Stuck, defined, 246
Subscribers in HMOs, percentage of, 4
Success, defined, 246
Suppliers, hospital satisfaction,
identification of, 24
Systems approach, to healing, 62

T

Tai Chi, 67
Taoist practice, 66–68
Targets, for visualization, 204
Technician, business behavioral style, 98
Technology, 27–34
business process, 30–34
computerization, 30–32
electronic data interchange, 31–32
Internet, 32
Intranet, 32
data sets, 32–34
clinical, 28–29
Telemedicine, 54–55
Telephone support, 55–56
Temperment awareness, 225–235
High-C—consciousness, 233–235
High-D—dominance, 227–228
High-I—influence, 229–231
High-S—steadiness, 231–233
personality, major spectrums of,
226–227

temperament awareness, 225–226
Thought field therapy, 69–70
Time management, 217–223
Time perspective, 171–172
Timeline
creation of, 191
transition and, 124–125
Training, 151–152
Transferable skills, identification of,
86–90
Transition, 121–129
stages of, 122–125

U

Union health insurance, hospital
satisfaction, identification of, 24

V

Value
corporate, 78–82
in health care, defined, 73–83
public perception of, 10–12, 82–83
Values, personal, 213
defined, 246
Vision, need for, 138–142
Visualization
mental, defined, 246
targets, 204
Volunteer organizations, networking
and, 240

W

Waveforms, series of, 77
Websites, 58
Workers' compensation, hospital
satisfaction, identification of, 24

About
the Authors

Michael Newell, RN, MSN, CCM, has 23 years of nursing experience, 15 in critical care and seven in case management. He is the author of *Using Case Management To Improve Health Outcomes* (Aspen Publishers, 1996). He is on the Board of Directors of the Professional Resource Network for Case Managers, the case management society of southern New Jersey, and the Delaware Valley Health Information and Management Systems Society.

Mario Pinardo is the president and founder of Achievement Dynamics Institute in Cherry Hill, New Jersey. His clients include Olympic athletes, sports teams, school districts, major corporations, and hundreds of professionals and small business owners. Over the last 12 years, he has delivered more than 2,400 workshops and seminars specializing in personal empowerment and increasing personal effectiveness.

You've read the book, now get the credit . . .

Interested in obtaining continuing education for *Reinventing Your Nursing Career: A Handbook for Success in the Age of Managed Care*? We'll mail you a free multiple-choice test packet. You choose whether to take a test for an individual chapter, multiple chapters, or the entire book. For a nominal price, you can earn contact hours at home. Discounts are available for multiple chapters or the entire book.

Call our corporate continuing education office at 1-800-866-0919 and request the *Reinventing Your Nursing Career* test packet today!

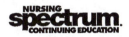

Nursing Spectrum is accredited as a provider of continuing education in nursing through the American Nurses Credentialing Center's Commission on Accreditation, by the State of Florida, Board of Nursing (provider no. 27I1768), and by the American Association of Critical-Care Nurses (96 01 07).